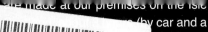

The Living Tree Orchid Es... ...are made at our premises on the isle
of Gigha in the Inner Hebrides in Argyll, ... (by car and a
brief ferry ride) from Glasgow. Arising w........ ...ach Flower
Remedies created by Dr. Edward Bach....... ....r essences
contain the subtle bio-electric healin........ ...water and
preserved with alcohol.

However, there are two principle dep....................... ....ng
Tree Orchid Essences (or LTOE for short). First o................ ...ms
or harm the plants in any way in order to make our essences. (.....er
description of this process will be found within this book.) Secondly, we choose
to work more or less exclusively with orchids, which we grow in a greenhouse
here on the island where we live. Nevertheless, the fundamental principles
are the same: that we are working with and exploring the gentle healing
energies of plants, expressed in their blooms & held in bottles of liquid.

What follows in the pages of this Guide are primarily my thoughts, knowledge
and recollections of experiences, as well as feedback from friends and our
(chiefly) therapist customers. I also describe the background of the LTOE which
were founded in the autumn of 1998, and address a number of questions relating
to the essences and their use. I hope that you will enjoy learning about and
experiencing the beauty and gentle power of the orchids.

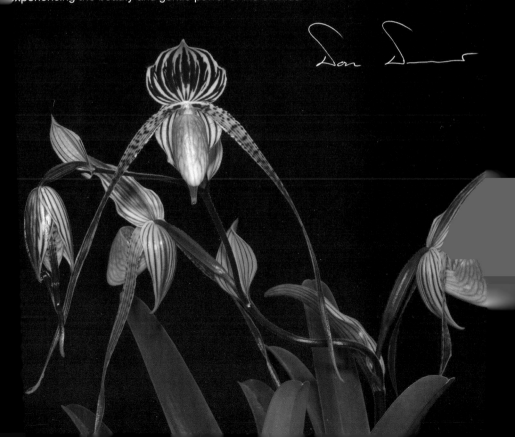

Foreword

I've had 40 years of experiences with the Bach flowers, and this has been in parallel with learning to recognise and express how I feel, and to be honest and brave enough to identify the negative sides of my nature. For me the journey has been (and IS) to cultivate and trust my intuition and etheric nature, and bring this into balance with the intellect. The Bach flowers are specific - angry, jealous - Holly; resentful, Willow; indecisive, Scleranthus, and so on... My work as an actor requires me to be aware and sensitive to changes of mood and emotion, and the flower remedies have been an enormous help to me in my career.

I was visiting Julie Bruton Seal for a herbal consultation, and was drawn to two blue wooden boxes on a shelf. There was somehow something more than symmetry, more than a pleasant colour; an unusually peaceful feeling I felt near them. Julie smiled when she saw my reaction to the boxes, and a little knowingly said "open it . . " Hard to put into words my feelings, impressions; it was like being in the presence of some One, some Essence, of great kindness and Knowing, of Healing; but also a hint of a map showing paths to Insight and Opening. I have the Orchid Essences now, and share them with my partner who experiences them directly and intuitively as she does with life. Mine is another voyage, a more linear and pragmatic approach, but one filled with the delight of discovery and the exciting prospect of more growth and Insight. We are Spiritual Beings undergoing a human experience - I sense these Essences can guide and assist us in that experience.

Martin Shaw

Norfolk, March 2010

Published in UK, March 2010
Copyright © Don Dennis ISBN 978-0-9542305-3-1
Published by International Flower Essence Repertoire, Achamore House
Isle of Gigha, Argyll, Scotland PA41 7AD
tel. 01 583 505 385

www.healingorchids.com

Designed by Don Dennis
Printed in the UK on Forest Stewardship Council certified paper
by David Jenkins Printing, Burnthouse Lane, Cowfold, West Sussex RH13 8DG England

Please note: the essences described in this book are not medicines.
They are not intended to cure or alleviate any medical condition.
If in doubt, always consult your normal medical practitioner.

In memory of Arthur Bailey
flower essence pioneer
and one of the finest men I have ever known

Introduction

Flower essences are used daily by hundreds of thousands of people around the world today. Primarily taking their inspiration from the work of Dr. Edward Bach (1886 - 1936), there are now several hundred essence makers around the world who are offering their products to the general public. Most people will have heard of the Bach Flower Remedies (which nowadays are made by a number of companies in Britain & Europe), while only a minority of people are aware that there are other ranges of flower essences available. Nevertheless in the UK many therapists are now familiar with the Australian Bush Flower Essences - at least in part thanks to the efforts of IFER to promote them almost since our inception in 1995. Very good quality essences from the USA, Canada, Brazil, France, Germany, Holland, India, New Zealand, Australia and elsewhere have appeared in the past 30 years, some with remarkable levels of research and application. In fact the Living Essences of Australia have some of their products being used in over 18 hospitals in the greater Perth region. And for better or worse, Dr. Bach's Rescue Remedy formula is now sold globally in many tens of millions of bottles each year.

Not Homeopathic

So what is in a bottle of a flower essence? The answer is both simple and subtle. Chemically speaking the only ingredients are water and alcohol - usually brandy, although we use organic French cognac. And this leads to some confusion, insofar as some people think that flower essences are a type of homeopathic product. This is quite definitely not the case, since flower essences are not prepared in the manner of homeopathic products. Homeopathic products involve multiple levels of both dilution and "seccussion". Seccussion is the vigorous shaking of the diluted liquid, and without this vital step one simply does not have a homeopathic preparation, since the seccussion is the means of creating the potency of the product.

Flower essences are not seccussed, and never need to be. They have just two levels of dilution from the "mother tincture", and no more. The first level of dilution is called "stock", and within the industry the second level of dilution is referred to as "dosage". In each of these states the liquid becomes progressively weaker as the dilution takes place. The opposite happens with homeopathic products. Homeopathy famously treats according to the principle of "like cures like" - and hence its name. Flower essences are not used in this way, with Dr. Bach himself declaring that his remedies treated illness on utterly different principles from homeopathy - a discipline with which he was deeply familiar.

What's in the Bottle?

So what is the active ingredient of a flower essence? It has variously been described as the etheric energy of the plant, or its Ch'i, or more plainly a bioelectric quality of the flower. Just as our bodies have a bio-electric structure*, so too do plants. And in making the mother tincture with a flowering plant, an essence-maker intends to impart into the waiting water something of this bio-electric quality from the blooms. I say "something" because we at present have no means of measuring the 'amount' of Ch'i which is imparted to the bowl of water, or indeed is imparted after one level of dilution (via a few drops of mother tincture) to the stock bottle. Of one thing though we can be certain: from the perspective of our everyday experience of electricity, the "something" will be a very minute quantity indeed. When it should happen that measuring apparatus becomes sensitive enough to detect the bio-electric component of a flower essence, we will probably be refering to units of picowatts or the like.

* Described in great detail by Chinese acupuncture over the past 3,000 years. Thankfully mainstream scientific research has begun to take place as well, though only in the past ten years has there been significant effort.

So How Can Essences Work?

A skeptical aquaintance once said to me that he couldn't give any credence to flower essences, as he could not imagine how such a miniscule charge of bio-electricity stored in the liquid could possibly have any effect on us. I finally realized after many months of pondering his statement that my most useful reply to this comment would be "Then just how much electricity do you think it takes for us to think a thought?"

The point of course is that our brains and nervous system clearly operate at the same level of subtlety as that found within the plant kingdom. It can hardly be otherwise, given the nature of our evolutionary co-creation. Photosynthesizing cellular life can be traced back in the fossil record about 3,000,000,000 years ago; complex multicellular life dates back slightly more than 1 billion years. Animals (as distinct from plants) only began appearing between 500 and 600 million years ago. It is generally reckoned that humans and chimpanzees emerged from a common ancestor between 5 and 7 million years ago.

Just how the animal kingdom emerged from a common ancestor with the plant kingdom is not for me to explore here, but the point is that before the two kingdoms divided, they had already developed the basic energy source and energy-utilization process (glycolysis & ATP) that is used by nearly all living things today. This process in itself has a bio-electric component, whether in a single-cell prokaryote or a rose bush or a human being. And so whatever unit of measure and description which is appropriate to the one organism, will be applicable to the rest. Given that the average power consumption of a human cell is just one picowatt (according to Wikipedia) it makes a great deal of sense that a few picowatts* of bio-electricity from a flower is able to have an effect on us.

The Mystery which is Water

The next question of course is, how is it possible for this bio-electric charge to be imparted to water? The answer is quite bluntly, we just don't know. Water is one of the most mysterious liquids we know of - and this is the view** of the scientific community, not simply a New-Age notion. But within the flower essence community water is nearly universally regarded as the best medium into which we can impart the energy of a flower. Humanity has a long tradition of using water in similar ways: think of Holy Water used in churches for example. In any case, a liquid is needed to hold the bio-electric energy, and long before Dr. Bach came on the scene in the 1930's announcing his remedies there have been people in various countries using water to make flower essences.

Bach & Before

I know directly of two essence makers who predate Dr. Bach. This is important to mention, as it is generally considered that Dr. Bach "invented" flower essence making. So to help set the record straight, here is a brief account of them.

Dr. Judy Griffin makes the (truly wonderful) Petite Fleur Essences in Texas, but her family emmigrated to the US from Italy. Judy's mother Flamina di Torrice made rose essences when Judy was a little girl; and her mother learned the skill from her mother Nunsadina Monzo. Nunsadina and her sister Antonio also made essences using snow from the nearby

*A picowatt is one-thousandth of a nanowatt, which is itself one-billionth of a watt. Ten square inches on Earth on a clear night apparently receives just under 7 picowatts of light from an average visible-light star.

** See the cover story of New Scientist magazine, Feb. 6th 2010: "The Strangest Liquid - Why Water is so Wierd" which describes a new theory of water's molecular structure.

mountains, where they lived near Salerno. A rose would be packed in some snow, and the melt-water would be given to people in the local village. They had learnt this technique from their mother Carmella Monzo, who was Judy's great-grandmother. Carmella would have been making her snow-rose essences in the Salerno area in the mid-1800's.

One of our long-term friends is a therapist named Syvia Kundrath, who divides her time between London and her native Austria, where she was largely raised by her grandfather Maximillian Ottowitz. Grandfather Max was a widely-read man, who in the course of his studies was inspired by the writings of Paracelsus (1493 - 1541) to make flower essences in the Carinthian Alps where he lived. He often used water from one of the local healing wells for this purpose, there being several such wells by the village of Maria-Elend where he lived. The blooms of *Euphrasia* (known locally as Augentrost) was a favourite of his for these purposes. Grandfather Max was born in 1884 and died in 1969, and Sylvia has read his journals dating back to before 1914 in which he describes the essence making process he was conducting. Max would not keep the essences for any length of time, and usually they were made for a person on that day - he would sense which flower would help them the most, and go out and make the essence.

So we have two very clear examples of essence-making* happening prior to Dr. Bach.

However the central importance of Dr. Edward Bach in the formation of what today may be described as the flower essence 'industry' cannot be over-stated. Nearly every flower essence maker in the world today is making their essences thanks to his pioneering work. And without the astonishing & self-effacing dedication of Nora Weeks, who looked after his work after his death until she passed away in 1978, we would quite likely not have heard of Dr. Bach.

Dr. Bach did three vital things to bring essences to the attention of the world. First of all, he wrote and spoke about his work, so that there is a body of writing to study, without which his work could easily have vanished. He also systematized his approach, so that any manner of emotional disturbances could be addressed via his remedies. And thirdly, he had the great insight that adding brandy to the water would help preserve an essence (whether mother tincture or stock) indefinitely. To my mind, this is the most important of his many contributions. It enables an essence made in Australia or California or Scotland to be sent halfway around the world, and be used perfectly well even several years after the bottling. What would otherwise have remained local folk medicine, has been able to develop much further, and even small cottage-industry essence makers are able to have a global audience for their essences.

Without the alcohol serving both to keep the water clear of bacterial and fungal growths, and also acting as a kind of anchor for the Ch'i of the flower, the wonderfully diverse market that exists today for essences would not be possible.

We are unable to say why or how alcohol acts as an anchor for the etheric energy of the plant, and this is one area where we must hope that eventually we will see some scientific research. Essence-makers would love to have a viable alternative, but to date we have seen no fully satisfactory alternative. Brandy, cognac and vodka each work very well for the purpose. A friend of mine has a set of Bach Remedies which are at least 50 years old, and the essences still have wonderful potency.

Another very interesting example is that of Tanmaya, who makes the Himalayan Flower Enhancers. He had never heard of the Bach Flower Remedies or of Dr. Bach, when he was guided by the flowers of the Himalayas in 1991 to make essences with them. Also, he makes his essences in alcohol rather than in water, as does Judy Griffin. Both quite separately had inner guidance to make them this way, and cited the same reason: to have a greater impact on the physical level.

Why Orchids?

With tens of thousands of flower essences being made in the world today (there are over 60 essence-making operations in the UK alone for example), surely there is little need for more..? It is true that there are many flower and other vibrational essences available now, and many of these are of a very high quality. But there are both special reasons for the making of essences with orchids, and also distinct challenges.

The family Orchidaceae represents nearly 10% of the flowering plants on Earth. There are some 800 genera, with very roughly 30,000 species. The vast majority of these are found in the tropics, although orchids are found on every continent except Antarctica. Because the vast majority of orchids are tropical, the typical amateur orchid grower tends to have an interest dominated by these plants. And it isn't simply the great number of species: there are also over 400,000 hybrids which humans have helped bring into being in the past 150 years.

The first person in the essence community to bring attention to the special qualities of orchids was Andreas Korte* of Germany, who pointed out in 1991 that orchid essences were able to have an effect on chakras that exist above our physical body - something which non-orchid essences are rarely able to do. Many others have made essences with orchids, but have simply included them in their overall range, without giving them particular focus. Star Riparetti of California has made a small range of essences with orchids found in the wild in Peru. The Alaskan Essences include a number of orchids amongst the 200+ flower, gem and environmental essences in their range. But it was Shabd-sangeet Khalsa (SSK) with her Dancing Light Orchid Essences who was the first person to make essences with orchids in a greenhouse, and then give these essences her principle focus. The passion she feels for orchids is powerfully expressed, and infectious. And so it was through her interest that I discovered my own.

However, to make essences with tropical orchids whilst living in the northern hemisphere pretty much necessitates having a greenhouse. That's the baseline requirement, as otherwise you are limited to what can fit and is willing to grow on your windowsills. (There are exceptions of course, but these tend to include reports of peeling wallpaper as the humidity climbs...) Beyond that you need the plants themselves, and as you begin a small collection, you will quickly find that such an interest is expensive! Beyond the realm of what is on offer in the supermarkets, there is a vast realm of beautiful diversity, and gone are the days when a single orchid might sell for the price of a house. The orchids I have bought over the years have cost on average just over £20 (roughly $30) each. That's not too bad, but when you have over 200 or 300 it quickly begins to challenge your bank balance.

Add to this the need to be obsessed, to be bitten by the orchid bug. Without that you simply will not have the inclination to devote countless hours looking after your plants on a daily basis year in and year out. I have been growing orchids for over a decade now, and must have spent close to 10,000 hours directly involved with caring for the orchids in my collection. It is not something to undertake lightly!

Beyond that there is a further requirement for orchid-essence making: some knowledge of

* IFER used to distribute Andreas' essences in the UK, and we hosted his Orchid Essence workshop twice in our early years. However, Andreas' interest was in the essences primarily, and not the orchids themselves, and so hosting his seminars did not awaken my interest in orchids. See our section "The People & The Story".

how to make a flower essence, and the impulse to do so. This may seem obvious, but these four things mentioned above rarely come together. There are an estimated 4 million amateur orchid growers in the world; there are at least the same number of people using flower essences, if not far more. There are at least 400 flower-essence makers worldwide today. Yet to the best of my knowledge, ours is the only company in the world since at least 2003 actively engaged in the making of essences with orchids as our primary focus.

And that seems a shame. One of the hopes I have in writing this book is to encourage others to consider making orchid essences, even if only as something to try for oneself. I believe that the flower essence community has the ability to describe an aspect of orchids that the orchid-growing community miss. You don't spend countless hours looking after orchids without having some sense of their beautiful mystery. But when orchids are approached only from a botanical standpoint, it is almost like admiring the work of Mozart by studying his music on paper, and never knowing it can be heard. There are utterly extraordinary qualities of orchids which I am convinced are able to be fairly readily experienced by way of taking drops of an orchid flower essence. And unless a person has a highly developed gift of sensing things unseen, then without the taking of the drops, that music, that tremendous unseen aspect of orchids will pass one by.

I have been a little "economical with the truth" in describing the active ingredient of essences as simply the bio-electric qualities of a flower. Within our field of work we generally regard what is held within the liquid in the essence bottle as to some degree the consciousness of the plant and flower. It is a living energy. I do not hold high hopes of a scientific explanation of this aspect of flower essence experience, given that the term "consciousness" is a contentious one within scientific circles. But the experience of both flower essence makers and therapists is that indeed these little bottles of water and alcohol seem to hold something of the living consciousness of the plant. And in the case of orchids, that consciousness is of a very high order.

What's in a Name?

Some years ago I met one of our good customers in the local supermarket. She had earlier been a frequent visitor to our premises in Sussex, but I hadn't seen her for two years. After greeting one another she explained that now she was well, so she didn't need the essences, and that was why she hadn't been in to see us for so many months. There was something about this comment that troubled me - and nothing to do with the lack of her making purchases. I knew that somehow my view of essences was at variance with the assumptions of her comment, yet I couldn't formulate my thinking around this with any clarity. It took a few more years for me to understand what was bothering me.

We generally regard the terms "flower essences" and "flower remedies" as equivalent, but they are not. A remedy is a product intended to help address a negative condition, in the way that Mimulus helps with fears of known things, or Crab Apple helps someone who suffers a sense of self-disgust. Dr. Bach specifically saw his essences as addressing remedial conditions of the psyche. But what if you are feeling fine, is there any role for flower essences when one is not feeling down, or guilty, or discouraged?

When Tanmaya of the **Himalayan Flower Enhancers** was meditating and fasting in the foothills of the Himalayas back in the early 1990's, he became so sensitive that he began to hear the flowers speak to him. After first wondering if he had gone mad, he found that they had very specific things that they wanted him to do: get a bowl, put a local high-grade alcohol

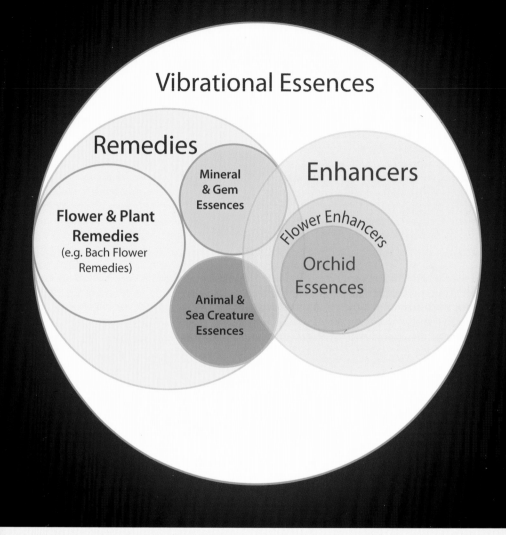

Vibrational Essences

Remedies

Mineral & Gem Essences

Enhancers

Flower & Plant Remedies
(e.g. Bach Flower Remedies)

Flower Enhancers

Orchid Essences

Animal & Sea Creature Essences

in the bowl, pick one of the flowers and float it in the bowl for some hours; and then eat the flower. He did as instructed, and found that the moment he ate the flower, he was flooded with information about the healing qualities of this essence.

Tanmaya had never been introduced to the Bach Flower Remedies at this point, being from rural Australia. But a friend gave him a book by Dr. Bach, after Tanmaya told her of his experiences with the flowers. And so he came to understand that what he had made were "flower remedies". He hiked back up to the foothills he knew and loved, and sat amongst the flowers again, who told him in no uncertain terms, "We are not remedies: we are not out to remedy anything! We are about enhancing fundamental soul qualities." And that is how his line got its name.

This story is of more than merely passing interest. We supply a great many kinesiologists from the UK and Europe with flower essences, and I had always been rather puzzled by the fact that certain ranges of essences I held in high regard were hardly ever specified by most of these kinesiologists. Then in 2003 I gave a talk to a large group of kinesiologists in London, and in the course of my talk I mentioned Tanmaya's story. The principle teacher, Richard Holding, picked up on this point about his essences not being remedies. He then created a hand-gesture for asking "Does this person need a flower enhancer?" And when he then tested this new question on a volunteer from the group, entire lines tested positive which had never tested positive for him before. The implication was clear: that whether he used the term essence or remedy, he had always meant "Does this person need a flower **remedy**?" And that was why Tanmaya's essences had never before been specified by him and his students, nor the Dancing Light Orchid Essences, nor our own Living Tree Orchid Essences.

So now the Venn diagram shown opposite can begin to make some sense. This diagram is as near as I can put into a visual format my thoughts on these distinctions within the realm of vibrational essences. Some essences are enhancers, and some are remedies. And some have aspects of both. So for example, in our own line, **Crown of Consciousness** is quite clearly an "enhancer", in that nobody walks around feeling bad because they are not having a full enough experience of their crown chakra...! On the other hand, **Angelic Canopy** is a terrific essence to use anytime that a person is feeling deeply upset or anxious; and yet it will help you to feel even better if you are already feeling fine. **Being in Grace** will help you to step into the dignity of the soul; but if you are holding onto toxic leftover emotions, it will help you to shed them. Then again, **Secret Wisdom** is one I would only ever take if I am intending to meditate, as it has a beautiful, silent depth it wishes to share.

Further notes for the Scientific Sceptic

This section is intended for the person who feels sceptical about flower essences on the premise that at present there can be found little in the way of scientific plausibility to the whole field of flower essences. I would like to say at the outset that I applaud your scepticism. Though I am not a scientist, I very deeply appreciate the rational spirit of science. And we in the field of flower essences can only lament the fact that there has been little by way of mainstream research into bio-electrics or other areas which might shed light on flower essences. There presumably is not much funding available from government departments or the military for programs of research into the ability of water to carry subtle bio-electric charges. Genetics and molecular biology is where the money is, and hence where the research is taking place.

And that has been the story ever since the 1940's with the entire field of bio-electrics. In the 1920's and 30's this was a field of great excitement and effort. Unfortunately, it became tainted by sloppy procedures and exaggerated claims. Then in the 1940's a distinguished biologist at the University of Chicago, Paul Weiss, announced that his research led him to conclude that electric fields had no effect on cells. This was an extraordinary and misguided pronouncement, effectively killing off research prospects in this area. And once Franklin, Watson & Crick discovered the double helix structure of DNA, more or less all biological research around the world then focused on molecular biology for decades ahead.

Until very recently, that was the way things stood. Today there is some interesting research taking place in the field of bio-electrics and even nanobioelectrics, but for the most part it is not looking in the directions we would need in order to give scientific substantiation to our field. However I feel confident that eventually there will be breakthroughs of both research and understanding that will confirm what flower essence therapists and makers have known all along: that there is a healing benefit for mind and bodies via the taking of drops of flower essences.

First Principles

There is a common fundamental problem with the scientific endeavour. It isn't fundamental to science, but is very common amongst scientists. This is the tendency to believe that the only things which exist in reality are those which science itself has been able to describe. Therefore anything which is posited beyond the current realm of scientific knowledge is regarded as likely to be insubstantial or a product of the imagination. To put it another way, science is only able to describe what it has been able to measure. And the limits of what we can measure is always and inevitably dictated by the limits of our technology. As our technology has improved, so has our ability to measure matter and the universe. But to imagine that the Large Hadron Collider will somehow be the ultimate tool for analyzing the pieces of the universe would be perverse. So long as there is continuous technological development, there will always be new abilities to measure the material universe beyond the level provided by the previous technological developments. Logically there can be no end to this; and as a result there can never be an end to new scientific knowledge and understanding.

We have known for a long time that there is a bio-electric structure to the body, and this is also to be found in plants. Bio-electricity has been a scientific topic since at least 1791 when Luigi Galvani published his research. But much of the research has concentrated on the mechanics of how our cells and nerves activate at the molecular level, rather than how communication at the intracellular level may in part take place via very weak electromagnetic fields. I am proposing that the reason that hundreds of thousands of people around the world swear by the benefits of flower essences, is because we require only a minute bio-electric charge from something for it to have an effect on our thoughts and our feelings, as I have discussed earlier.

Furthermore, there are two basic tenets of our industry which should be capable of being verified, if not at the moment, then in the very near future. The first is the assertion that water is capable of briefly holding some very small electrical charge, a charge which would probably be measured as fluctuations at the picowatt level. The second assertion is that somehow the molecular nature of alcohol is such that it acts to hold that electric charge within the water, when mixed in a 50-50 ratio. If flower essences were sold without alcohol mixed in, the energy of the flower would dissipate prior to being bought by the end-user. The accepted view within our industry is that, so long as a bottle of a flower essence has at least 50% brandy (= 20% alcohol) then that bottle will still have the bio-electric energy of the flower for at least 10 years. So with the right equipment, these two working notions of our industry should be very readily examined. Whether such equipment exists, or will be able to be developed in the near future, I have no idea. But such research would be of great interest to everyone involved with flower essences.

Given that a good FM radio can pick up a signal of as little as a few femtowatts (femtowatt= one thousandth of a picowatt), we may have cause to be optimistic that within a few years there may be sensors capable of measuring fluctuations of picowatts in liquids. And yet there is already an instrument of more than sufficient sensitivity to detect the minute bio-electric charges of flower essences: the human brain and nervous system.

That is why I prefer to encourage people to go beyond discussion, to use a clear and simple method for discovering the validity to the claims of the flower essence community: try it and see. This in effect is what is at the core of the Scientific Method. Scepticism is fine, so long as it prevents gullibility; but it should not be a barrier to reflection and exploration. Unfortunately, much of the language we use to describe essences is a barrier to the scientific sceptic. But then the layman experiences a similar barrier when encountering the specialist use of language in scientific journals. This is the nature of how groups use language. Try to get past the language barrier, suspend judgement briefly, to allow the other point of view the opportunity to explain itself. We have to overcome our own prejudices and preconceptions if we are to develop bridges of understanding. And it behooves us to bear in mind that it is often through such efforts at inter-group communication that the most significant breakthroughs are able to take place, to everyone's benefit. It is all very well to have a good dialogue within your professional peer group, but such dialogue is not necessarily the most fertile ground for new insights arising.

Some 8 or 9 years ago I met an outstanding biochemist from University College London. He was clearly very, very good within his chosen discipline. We discussed our new orchid essences, which he admired. He told me he couldn't explain how they worked, but that they did work he was quite certain. He had tried them. Of course, he said to me, he couldn't come out in any public way to make such a statement, or his funding prospects would shrivel up. "Look", he said, "there's a great deal we very simply do not understand. Just because we cannot yet explain a phenomena, is not a reason to dismiss it." I liked his attitude, and I wished him well.

In my student days, a Trustee of my school had a dialogue with me about my interests while at the school. He was a theoretical physicist of some note, and he simply said to me that "The most important endeavour while at school is to attempt to grasp the spirit of Reason". I have done my best to hold to that principle in my life, and in my reflections on things. And my work with the orchid essences, though endlessly filled with awe at their beauty and mystery, is also guided by that notion.

Making Orchid Essences

If you grow orchids, you will know that it can be a long wait sometimes to see a particular plant come into bloom. In some case this can be a matter of years. And when the blooms appear, the majesty of the bloom is astonishing. It is perhaps at this point that the wish to find a means to make a flower essence without having to cut the bloom becomes most poignant. Though I know several essence-makers who have cut orchids to make essences, I cannot countenance the idea myself. There simply is no need to cut an orchid if you wish to make an essence; and in my view, it will be a more vibrant essence, if the plant has not been cut or otherwise harmed.

Vasudeva and Kadambi Barnao of the Living Essences of Australia call their range Living Essences for the simple reason that they do not cut the blooms, but rather pour water over the living blooms (out in the wild) into a catchment bowl. Andreas Korte has his own method too*, though it is not one we use. And SSK with her Dancing Light Orchid Essences simply places a bowl of water underneath the orchid bloom for a few hours, in order to make her essences. The Shahs in Mumbai, who make the Aum Himalaya Sanjeevini Essences also make most of their essences without cutting the flowers. So there are many examples around the world of good quality flower essences being made without resorting to cutting the blooms in the manner of Dr. Bach's sun-bowl method.

Our basic technique is illustrated and outlined on the following pages. But if you wish to make an orchid essence, let the orchid call you, feel in your heart a certain pull, like it is knocking loudly on the door of your mind, asking you to involve it in the essence-making. You will find better results if that call from the orchid is there. Though the steps are simple and clear, the process is certainly not merely a technical process. There is an inward process of spirit, between you and the orchid, which also must be at play in this.

The Korte method involves holding a bowl of water in one's hand directly under the bloom for a few minutes. However we prefer to minimise the time in which we are near to the bowl, the water and the orchid, to ensure the least possible 'contamination' of the essence with our own energies.

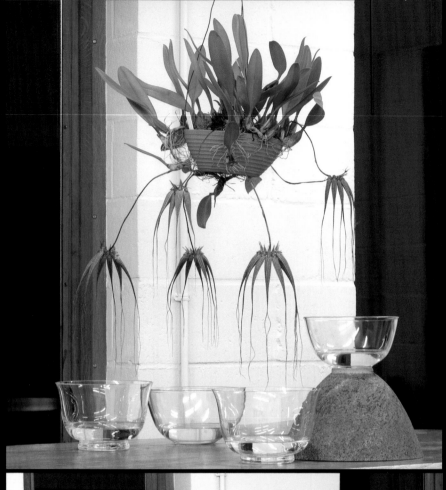

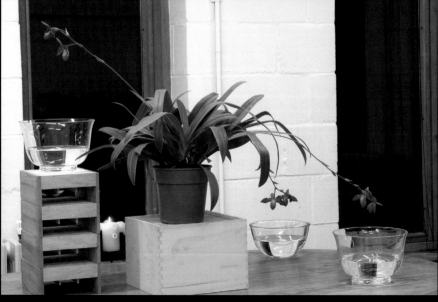

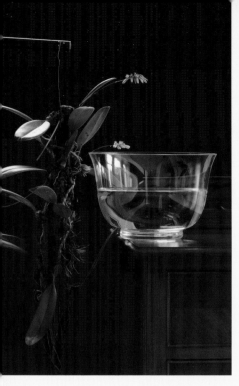

Essence-Making

Our essence-making is predicated on a few simple principles. First of all, we do not want to either cut or harm the orchid or its bloom. Secondly, as the orchid has been living inside a greenhouse, it seems sensible to make the essence indoors. (And in fact much of the year it would be too cold outside for the orchid.) Thirdly, we want as little of our own energy as possible to be in the essence. And lastly, we want only the one orchid's energy in the essence, hence it cannot take place readily within the greenhouse itself.

Therefore the room we use for essence-making is cleansed both physically and energetically, and is undisturbed for the duration of the making. We have to be in the space only at the beginning in order to arrange the orchid and the bowl or bowls of water; and to come into the space at the very end, to pour the water over the bloom or blooms. But otherwise the space becomes the temple of that orchid during the hours of the essence forming.

Here is our procedure in ten clear steps.

1. Cleanse the space.

2. Quieten the mind and heart.

3. Bring the orchid into the space.

4. Set up the bowl(s) of water under the blooms.

5. Leave the space undisturbed, usually between 6 and 24 hours.
   Electric lights *must* be turned off.

6. Then quietly enter the space, be still a couple of minutes, well away from the orchid.

7. Gently pour a bit of water from the bowl(s) over the blooms.

8. Add brandy in equal measure to the water (i.e., a 50/50 ratio) in the bowl(s).

9. Pour this Mother Tincture into large glass bottles for storage.

10. Sip the last teaspoon of the Mother Tincture. Sit, be still.

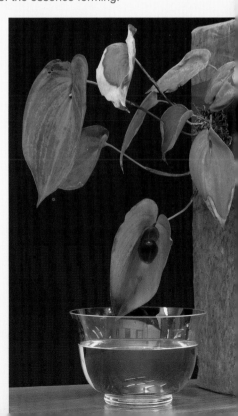

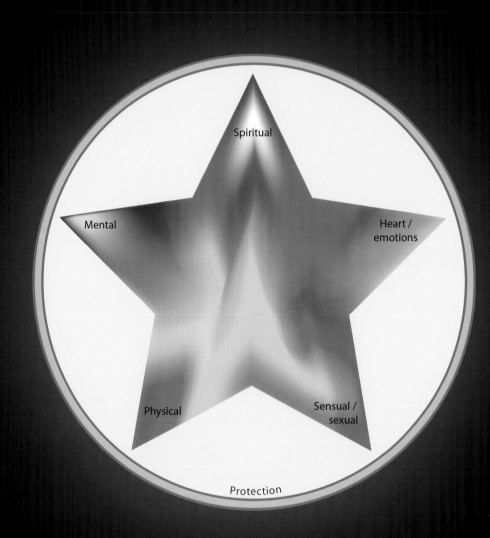

Getting to Know the Essences

If one wishes to learn about the writings of Plato, would you prefer to hear what Professor Smith has to say on the topic, or read Plato's writings themselves? In a similar manner, the best way to get to know the LTOE is to try them, to take a few drops and sit quietly for ten or 15 minutes, to see what effects you feel. To a large degree this is the approach I use in the seminars I teach, though I will also share much of our shared understanding of the qualities of each essence. But no amount of verbal information can replace the value of directly experiencing the energies of the orchids via their essences.

For those who are relatively new to essences, or for those who have a deep background with essences but for whom the LTOE are new, I would wish to emphasize the merit of this approach. This can be done at home, as long as you can take a little time out and have a tranquil space without fear of interruption. To get a few friends or colleagues together once a week or once a month of an evening, and meditate on 3 or 4 essences together is a good approach too, as then each person's experience can be shared, and a broader perspective of the essence is arrived at. If a group gets together, it helps to have one person act as the moderator for the sharing after each meditation.

In the seminar I teach, we move in a certain progression through the essences, more or less in keeping with the points of the star shown opposite. Beginning with those essences with the greatest impact on a physical level (e.g., **Internal Cleansing**, **Renewing Life**, **Settling with a Smile**) we then over the days of the seminar meditate on the ones with some degree of focus on the sensual/sexual side of our being; then the ones addressing primarily the heart and emotions; then the mental level. At some point we also experience those essences which help us to protect ourselves, such as **Soul Shield** and its constituent elements. Only after moving through this progression of the essences do we then try the essences in the range which have an almost purely spiritual focus. It is a bit like climbing higher and higher into the mountains, and acclimatising as one goes up. That way, by the time you reach the snowy peaks, you are able to breathe the rarified air more readily. In seminars it is often commented on the final day that the participants are glad they only got to **Crown of Consciousness**, or **Behold the Silence**, or **Secret Wisdom** at the end, that the previous days meditations on the other essences was necessary for the deeper appreciation of the very fine energies of these last ones.

Of course there is great value (I hope!) in reading what we can share about the essences, otherwise this book could serve little purpose. But one must always remember, the words are not the essence. Nothing is a substitute for directly experiencing the essences, preferably whilst one is sitting quietly so that the inner senses can note the subtle inner processes and shifts the essences bring about. Particularly for the therapist there is a further value in having the essences be known at some level by your own body directly: it will assist your work with clients in several respects. First of all, the essence(s) your client will benefit from especially is likley to come to mind readily once you have the orchids' energies 'under your skin' as it were. You will also be able all the better to sense the shifts that the essence brings about in the client. And you will be healing your own spirit at deep levels, and finding inspiration through the process of getting to know the orchid essences in this meditative way.

It is very good to augment that process by studying the photos of each orchid, which is both one of the purposes of this book, and also of our website (www.healingorchids.com) and of our set of orchid photo cards - but more on those later.

Why Gigha?

IFER had been based since its inception in southern England, in the building we called The Living Tree. In the days when I was running a small timber business there, dealing with sustainably-managed hardwoods (our sawmill business helped found the Forest Stewardship Council or FSC, which is recognized today as the primary valid logo for responsibly-harvested timber products worldwide) we called the premises The Working Tree. Two years after IFER began, SSK visited to teach a seminar, and recommended that we change the name of the building to The Living Tree, to reflect the fact that we were now dealing in flower essences rather than timber. That felt right, and that's how it came to be that our building got its name. And so in turn that is how The Living Tree Orchid Essences got their name.

As fine as our premises were, and tucked away in a lovely Sussex valley, there was nevertheless one serious limitation it presented: we couldn't host residential seminars. Flower essences need a lot of educational input to help people know how to work most effectively with them, and to that end we had hosted many dozens of workshops and seminars both at the Living Tree and

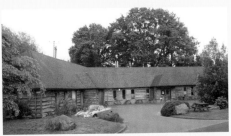

elsewhere over a period of eight years. But these were almost invariably two-day workshops at weekends, and I realized that it would be very valuable for the flower essence community if we were in a position to offer longer residential seminars where the topics could be explored in greater depth. And as my three children had moved up to Edinburgh with their mother after she and I had divorced, it came about that I found myself looking in Scotland for suitable premises.

I had a tall order: I needed a house which I could afford (by selling The Living Tree) and which was large enough to enable at least 18 guests to stay for up to a week. Clearly I would need to run the house as a B&B in between seminars, to pay the mortgage. Looking around estate agents websites for several days I could find nothing suitable which I could afford, and so gave up on the idea entirely. Then one month later, in June 2003, I was reading one of the Sunday papers when I came upon a large article about a large old house up for sale by the community which just 15 months previously had bought their island off the last laird. And for various reasons, especially the island location, the asking price for the house was not far beyond what I reckoned were my means once the Living Tree was sold. I flew up within a few days to have a look, and I went back up to Gigha twice in July to look again. I had to be vetted by a committee of the community, and then later I made a presentation to most of the community. My offer was made (and accepted) in August, and I moved up to this small island in the Inner Hebrides in December 2003.

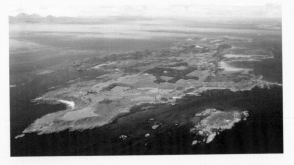

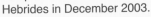

The Isle of Gigha is roughly 6 miles long and one mile wide, and has about 150 residents. At the time of the community buy-out in March 2002 the population was down to just 98, and there were just 6 pupils in the local primary school. As of early 2010 there are now 25 pupils, which is just one of the measures of success of the buy-out. For those folk not familiar with land ownership in Scotland, I will just mention that Scotland has been the last hold-out of feudal land ownership in the whole of Europe, such that roughly 90% of the land of the country is owned by a small number of families. The Isle of Gigha had gone through a succession of owners since 1880, some good and others less so. In

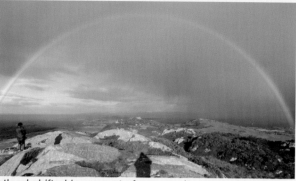

the 1990's the political climate in Scotland shifted in support of community ownership where possible in such cases as Gigha, and so when the last laird chose to sell, the residents of Gigha had the necessary political support at the national level to enable the community buy-out to happen.

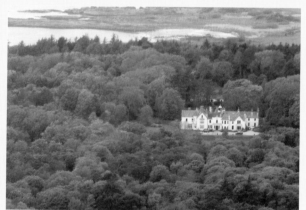

However as part of the complex arrangements of support provided for the buy-out, a substantial sum had to be repaid to the Scottish Land Fund by March 2004. As part of the needed fund-raising efforts, the community trust put Achamore House up for sale, and that was how I came to have the opportunity to buy it and relocate myself and IFER up to this beautiful island.

It only takes one visit to Gigha to see why many visitors return again and again over the years. Although it is off the beaten tourist track (think Arran, or Islay, Iona and Oban) yet this island is exceptionally blessed with the rugged beauty of the Hebrides. There are 4 dairy farms working most of the agricultural land, and an offshore fish farm, and an award winning onshore fish farm. Go around the coast of Gigha by boat to see the stunning scenery of the western shore rocks, or the magical island of Cara just south of us. Take walks over many days without seeing the same path twice, or ride a bicycle to the north end and back. And then several times a year there will be dances ("Ceilidh") in the nearby Village Hall, open to all. It is a friendly island, and visitors are made to feel very welcome.

And then there are the gardens surrounding Achamore House. Created by Col. Sir James Horlick and his lover Kitty Lloyd-Jones beginning in 1944, the 52 acres of rhododendrons, azaleas and camellias of Achamore Gardens are their greatest legacy to the island. They also provide a wonderful setting for our flower essence seminars. I believe that anyone visiting Achamore House will understand immediately why I felt it was right to make the move up here!

Seminars

The principle purpose of the move to Gigha was in order to have premises and a location suitable for longer, residential seminars. And to this end the move was highly successful. As IFER carries about 18 other lines of essences from around the world, we host seminars taught by the various makers, as long as there is sufficient interest. We have hosted Sabina Pettitt of the Pacific Essences twice since the move to Gigha, each seminar being about a week long.

Tanmaya of the Himalayan Flower Enhancers has taught week-long seminars here twice. Steve Johnson from Alaska taught at Achamore House twice, again with week-long seminars. And we hosted two small flower essence gatherings here as well, with many of the various essence-makers we represent coming for these 4-day events. I am especially pleased that Christine Bailey & her late husband Arthur came to both of our mini-conferences, and indeed Arthur made two essences here in Achamore Gardens - his **Flame Azalea** and **Conifer Mazegill** essences.

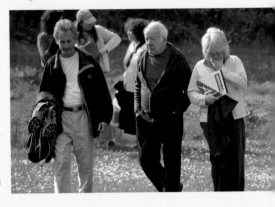

Our old friend David Carson also has been to Gigha twice, teaching about the Native American spirit medicine of which he is so deeply knowledgable (see his books **Medicine Cards**; **Crossing Into Medicine Country**; and **Oracle 2012**). David's daughter Greta accompanied him on both trips here, and very much shared in the teaching of the workshops.

Peter Tadd also taught a week-long seminar at Achamore, saying afterwards it was "the best workshop he'd ever taught". We tend to favour 6 or 7 day workshops, as it does take most people the best part of a day to travel here, and we wish to make that journey worthwhile.

Everyone has appreciated how safe and nurturing an environment is provided here at Achamore House, augmented no end by the sheer beauty of the gardens and the island.

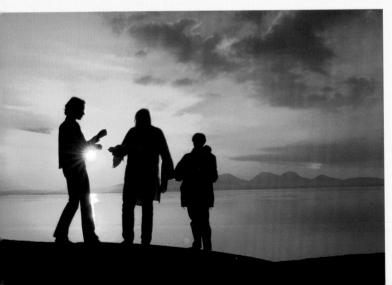

Of course, the seminars which are taught by folk who have to travel great distances to get here, and who also have to take that week out of their schedule back home, are by necessity somewhat expensive - all the more so because the seminars tend to have an upper limit of about two dozen people attending.

I came to realize that it made a great deal of sense for me to offer several seminars a year here on our orchid essences. There are five main reasons for this:

1. I need to be here anyway, looking after the orchids in the greenhouse. The orchids require daily care, and it isn't easy to explain to others all the nuances of care that the 50+ genera require.

2. I don't like traveling all that much.

3. There is the demand, fortunately!

4. By teaching here, the attendees get to meet the orchids themselves, and spend some time in the greenhouse.

5. As I am already here, and the house is run as a B&B, we are able to keep the cost of a week-long seminar taught by me down to a minimum.

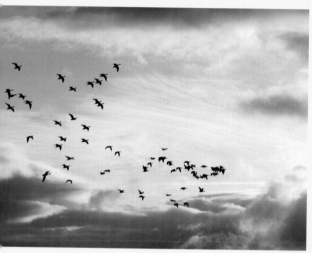

In Sussex we used to host seminars for certain developers which had as many as 90 people attending. And that can work if the seminar is simply about sharing information about what each essence can be used for etc. But the approach I take is very different, as indicated earlier: I want people to take each essence (more or less) over the course of the 6 days.

We also allow a day for seeing the island, exploring Gigha's lovely beaches, and may go out by boat, with a chance of seeing dolphins - see the following pages photos.

We meditate as a group on each essence in turn, and we share our experiences with one another after each meditation*. In order to maintain a high quality of sharing, the seminar is limited to just 10 participants. And I have found this works well. There is the extra 'reward' for me of having the opportunity to spend another week communing with the orchids again!

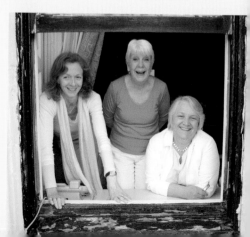

* I am using the word meditation here in a very general, and definitely non-religious sense. There is no technique to meditating on an orchid essence: I simply mean we sit quietly with our eyes closed, and see if we are able to sense the gentle impact of a given essence.

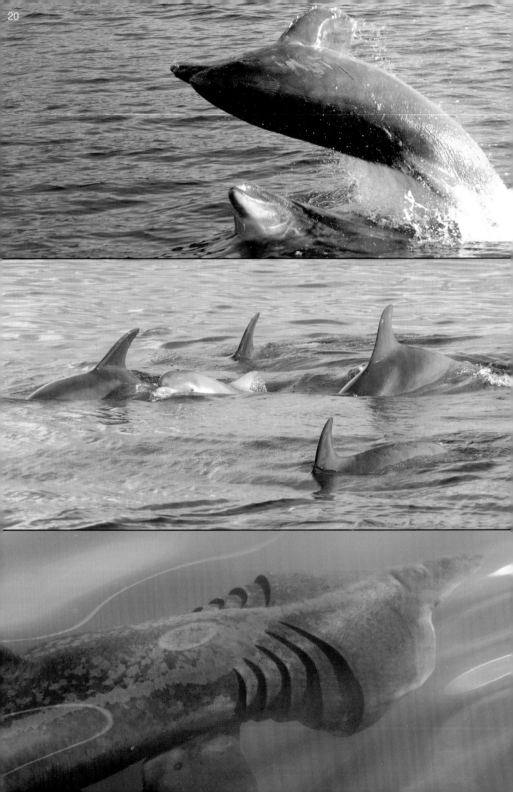

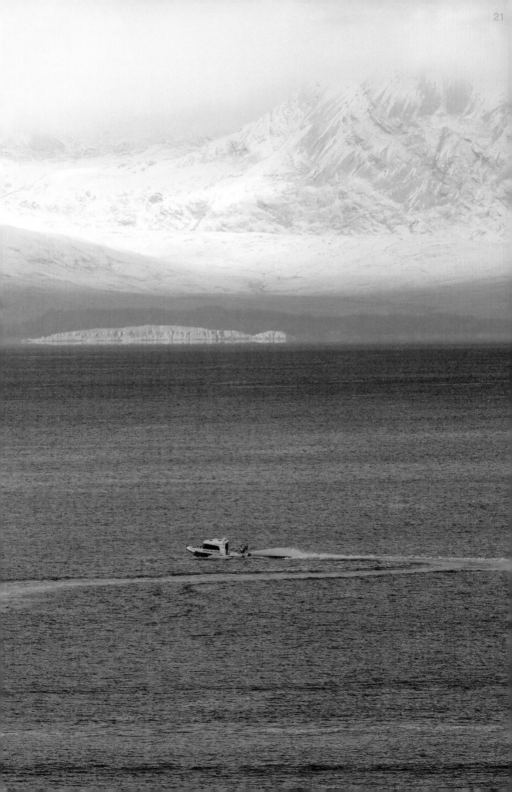

The People & the Story

The development of a project of this nature always requires a good number of people, both those directly and indirectly involved. There are several people about whom I can safely say the LTOE would not have been created were it not for their input or involvement.

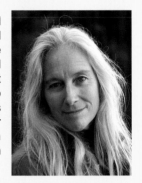

First of all, my passion for orchids came about by being introduced to them by Shabd-sangeet Khalsa of the Dancing Light Orchid Essences (DLOE). I met her at the International Flower Essence Conference held at Findhorn in October 1997. At this point she had been making essences with orchids grown in greenhouses for just under a year, with Carson Barnes (a commercial orchid grower who has what appears to be encylopaedic knowledge of orchids, and is based near San Francisco, CA). SSK (as she is known to her friends) had previously been making flower essences in the Alaskan wilderness for some 18 years, where she co-founded the Alaskan Flower Essence Project with Steve Johnson.

As far as I am aware, prior to 1996 nobody had ever made an essence with a greenhouse-grown orchid. SSK was herself reluctant to do so at first, as she had always made her flower essences in the wilderness, or occasionally in her large garden. But in her contact with the orchids in their greenhouse, their communication with her was so insistent and determined, in effect (as she describes it) *demanding* that she make essences with them, that her range of essences came into being. When I tried her essences at the Findhorn Conference, I was astonished at their potency and depth - I had not encountered essences like this before. We

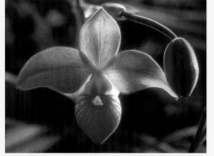

agreed that IFER would be the importer/distributor in Europe for the DLOE, and after dropping her off at Heathrow shortly after the conference, I stopped off at the garden centre at RHS Wisley and bought an orchid. In the months that followed, that little slipper orchid captured my interest and my affection. It grew rapidly once SSK told me it needed frequent watering. And when it came into bloom again in early autum 1998, I had an extraordinary experience with *Phragmipedium Hanne Popow*.

I was watering the orchid late one night, and as I placed her back on the window sill, I very distinctly heard the orchid say, "Make an essence with me." I was rather shocked. My recollection is that I spoke out loud back to 'her', saying "You've got the wrong guy, I'm an essence **distributor**, not an essence maker." (In the years since this experience, I have only ever 'heard' an orchid on two or maybe three other occasions. Usually I will simply feel the orchids with my heart.) The communication from the orchid was experienced by me as words I heard in my head, and utterly distinct from the thoughts I had going through my mind at the time. And apart from being surprised to hear an orchid speak, I had firmly decided some months before that night that I was more suited to the role of being an essence importer/distributor than an essence maker - hence my retort.

My old friend Peter Tadd visited a few days later, to give a talk on his clairvoyant work. After everyone had left that evening, I showed *Phrag. Hanne Popow* to Peter, and told him of my experience. To him it was obvious that the orchid wanted me to make an essence with her, and when I queried that, he said that it was due to the heart-felt connection I had with the plant.

She also wanted it to be set up that night, though Peter didn't know why. So I took Peter back to the cottage I lived in, and then went back to the Living Tree and set a bowl of water under the bloom in the manner I had been shown by SSK. After 'tuning in' to the orchid, I then went home for the night.

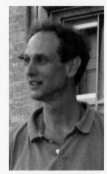

In the morning, Peter and I went to look at the orchid and the bowl of water. By SSK's technique, I had done all that was needed. But Peter commented that there was a lot of light "hovering over the water, but not *in* the water". I mentioned how the Living Essences of Australia are made, by pouring water over the blooms into a catchment bowl. Peter reckoned that ought to help. So I fetched a little clean beaker from the kitchen while Peter wandered around the shop, and I then dipped it into the water in the bowl, and poured this very gently over the blooms, back into the bowl. I then found Peter to have him 'cast his 3rd eye' on the matter, and he said "Yep, that's done it." The light from the orchid was now in the water. So I then added brandy in equal measure to the water, and decanted it into a few large glass bottles, and the first essence was born.

Peter and I discussed the properties of this essence in the hours that followed, and by evening we had a pretty clear understanding of not only what it would help with, but also why the orchid had wanted it set up that night. That this orchid should convey qualities of affection and a loving heart is fairly obvious to anyone either taking the essence, or looking at the photo of it. But the timing of the making had ensured that during most of the hours the essence was forming, a bud also was opening into bloom. What had been a closed bud when I left it that night, was a fully open bloom 9 hours later in the morning. (I have observed since that it takes Phrag. Hanne Popow about six hours to open her buds, so our timing was fairly extraordinary.) So if you can understand that this orchid conveys loving affection, yet for several hours while the 2nd bloom was opening, this second bloom was reflecting that loving energy back within herself. And so the very important second quality of this essence is to help us love ourselves, for the affection of our hearts to nurture ourselves, as well as those around us.

I made a number of orchid essences in the year that followed. Somewhere in this period I also got bitten by the orchid bug, and went to several orchid shows in England, and to a few commercial orchid establishments. Soon I had too many orchids for all the windowsills at the Living Tree, and before long I had a lean-to greenhouse built at the back of the premises. Initially I bought only phragmipediums, but gradually my interest broadened, and then the

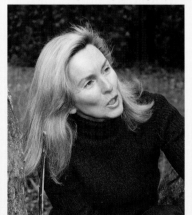

floodgates opened. In the five or six years that followed, I bought in excess of 800 orchids. This is not something I would recommend... It is not uncommon though amongst people who get the orchid bug. It is difficult to explain the fascination these plants hold for those of us who grow them, and spend our resources as well as endless hours looking after them.

However, it is very likely that my essence-making would have remained a low-key personal activity, had it not been for our friend Heather DeCam entering the picture. Heather and her husband live not far from our former premises, and she had been buying essences from IFER since the end of 1996. As it happened, Heather was the first person we gave this first orchid essence to try, other than ourselves. She 'got' the essence very readily and without prompting. But she had no other involvement with the orchid essences at that point. I occasionally made an essence with one of the orchids that came into bloom, a few of which are in the line today. But in January 2000 Heather visited our shop the Living Tree one day, and I showed her the orchids in the greenhouse. There was one in particularly fine bloom, a *Phragmipedium Saint Ouen*.

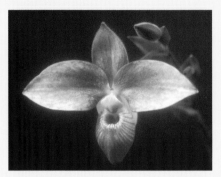

Two days later Heather called me to ask if I was going to make an essence with that lovely orchid. I explained to her that much as I would like to, my days that month were a bit too stressful to think of having the right conditions for essence-making. I well understood by this point that in effect essence-making is what I call a "temple activity": that you need to be able to get into a fine, clear and stress-free frame of mind and heart as otherwise the essence will inevitably reflect your stress to some degree. But Heather told me that each night when going to bed she had seen the blooms of Phrag. St. Ouen appearing very clearly before her. She commented that she too was experiencing some stress in her life, but she had the feeling that perhaps this orchid would be able to help both of us at that point.

I told Heather that the only way I could see making an essence that weekend would be if she were to come over to the Living Tree and help me with the process. By this point Heather was already the sort of good friend who lightens your spirits as soon as you see them, so I knew that it would be alright if she participated. She agreed to do so, but what happened was very unexpected. Not only was the essence-making stress-free, but somehow it was simply and utterly delightful. I can only liken it to the difference between dancing by yourself, and dancing with a partner. But Heather brought a special quality to the process which I would struggle to describe. Something high and very fine, and her presence seemed to refine the space of the room where the essence-making took place. (By this point, we had a room at the far end of the premises that was used for essence-making, and very little else. Far from any hustle and bustle and noise, it was an ideal spot for the process.) And so the essence called Golden Radiance was brought into being.

A few weeks later there was another orchid I felt it would be good to make an essence with, and I called Heather to ask if she would like to help once again. She said yes, again it was sheer delight, and in the next 46 months we ended up making 39 orchid essences together. It is very clear to me that our range of the Living Tree Orchid Essences would not have come into being without Heather's involvement. While SSK inspired my interest in orchids, and pioneered the idea of making essences with orchids growing in greenhouses; and while Peter Tadd provided important feedback about them, it was Heather's role in the making of the essences themselves that was key to the formation of the line. Without Heather's involvement, there would be no Living Tree Orchid Essences today, of this I feel certain.

In those early years of the essence-making at the Living Tree, there were also two young members of staff who came to participate in the essence-making with us. Natalie Shaw's mother Gail had been our very first member of staff, she having been a flower essence therapist for many years prior to 1996, and consequently brought valuable knowledge and skills to IFER. In due course both of her two daughters Francine and Natalie came to work at the Living Tree. Each had a deep understanding of essences, having been raised with them.

I showed Natalie one of the orchids in bloom in the greenhouse one day in early February 2002, a *Scaphosepalum swertifolium*. That night the orchid appeared in a dream to Natalie, very clearly. When she told me her dream, I knew straight away that we would need to make an essence with this orchid, as this would be the best way for Natalie to receive its wisdom. And so it made a great deal of sense that Natalie should be involved in the essence-making, on at least this occasion. And that was how the essence Life Direction (Lanata) was brought into being. I made the essence with Natalie, both so she could be shown the whole process which Heather and I had developed by this point, and so there would be a yin-yang framework for the making. Over the next few years, Natalie and I made a total of five essences together.

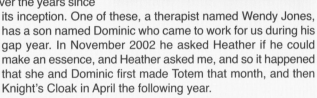

IFER has been blessed with many wonderful and often extraordinary customers over the years since its inception. One of these, a therapist named Wendy Jones, has a son named Dominic who came to work for us during his gap year. In November 2002 he asked Heather if he could make an essence, and Heather asked me, and so it happened that she and Dominic first made Totem that month, and then Knight's Cloak in April the following year.

The making of the latter was especially interesting to me, as it came about after I had been watering and caring for the orchid (*Pleurothallis gargantua*) for about 18 months. Another essence-maker Rose Titchiner of the Light Heart Essences (in Norfolk, England) had been visiting our premises, and saw this remarkable orchid (shown here below right, in detailed close-up) in bloom. Later, she spoke with Dominic by phone about it, and this was how Dominic ended up suggesting to Heather that perhaps they should make an essence with this orchid that had so caught the eye of Rose. I am grateful to Rose for having brought the orchid in our greenhouse to Dom's attention! (An essence made by Rose - Child's Play - is also a component of our latest combination, Sacral Regulator.)

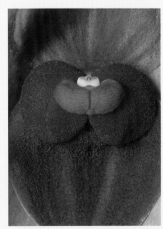

In December 2003 I relocated our business from the south of England to a small island in the Inner Hebrides in Scotland. This was, as you may imagine, a fairly major upheaval. The move was right and a deeply good thing to do, but it was not without its sacrifice. The hardest part of the move for me was knowing that Heather and I would only rarely meet up, and even less often have the opportunity to make further essences together. Nevertheless, we stay in touch, and usually meet up at least once a year.

In the first period after the move to Gigha, I didn't have a greenhouse, and as a consequence I had to give many of the orchids away to friends down south. Several dozen moved up here with me, but conditions were not ideal until I was able to build a greenhouse here beside Achamore House. This greenhouse is 27 feet long, and about 10 feet wide, and as of January 2010 houses a fine collection of over 700 orchids, the great majority of which are species. To have the chance to not only see the orchids, but also to experience their energies first-hand, is one of the primary reasons that I rarely travel elsewhere to teach about the essences. The experience for people who take the trouble to travel here to attend the orchid essence seminars is far richer than could possibly be the case away from our greenhouse.

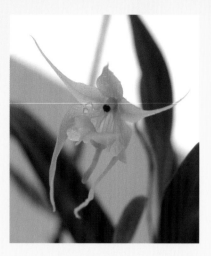

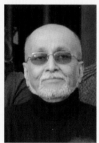

One of our long-standing therapist customers, who has been to Gigha several times, and who of late has been making significant contributions to the development of the LTOE range, is Dr. Adrian Brito-Babapulle. Originally from Sri Lanka, Adrian has lived in the UK for the past 40 years, and has an extraordinary number of academic and professional qualifications to his name. But it is in his work over the past decade in developing a deep form of kinesiology where he has found special ways of working with our orchid essences, which are the core of his 'energy toolbox'. On his visits in the past two years, Adrian has found himself powerfully drawn to certain orchids in the greenhouse, with this leading to us making several essences either together, or my making them on my own but at his instigation. (Sometimes the instigation comes from me, but who does the instigating isn't that important. What is important is that either of us are in effect responding to the orchid, sensing its call as it were. If I were to simply randomly choose an orchid to make an essence with, the resulting essence would be lacking. The 'call' of the orchid is important, as this is a kind of peak energetically in the orchid's cycle of being to which we are responding.)

A good illustration of our process at work is with the essence Shadow Warrior. In the autumn of 2007 while browsing orchid websites, I came across an image of this extraordinary species of the genus Bulbophyllum, which is the largest of the genera in the family orchidaceae. I contacted one of the very fine semi-commercial orchid growers I know, a fellow named Malcolm Perry who is based near Bristol. I asked him if he knew where I could get ahold of a *Bulbophyllum phalaenopsis*. He reckoned he did, and some months later, brought a fine specimen back

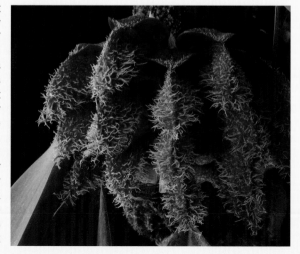

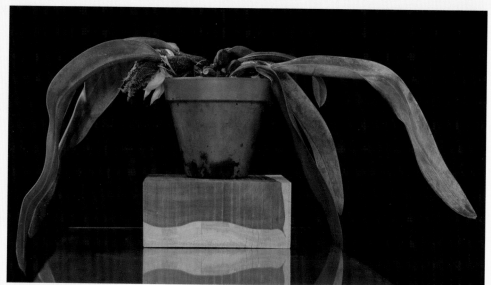

from Germany for me. My intuition had said that this was an important orchid for us to work with. Then in the summer of 2008 Adrian visited when this orchid happened to be in bloom. He first addressed his attention to the orchid which produced the essences Healing the Higher Heart & Spirit of the Higher Heart. Then on the following day when he went into the greenhouse, the *Bulbo. phalaenopsis* simply grabbed his attention. He said to me that he had been looking for years for an essence that would do what this orchid's essence would achieve, in helping to address our shadow aspect. And so Shadow Warrior was born.

Adrian's work with the orchid essences has been fascinating to observe as it has developed, with the energetic possibilities presented by the orchids bringing about deeper levels of reach in his kinesiology, and his kinesiology bringing us to seek certain qualities amongst the orchids. In later pages in this book Adrian describes in outline the nature of his approach.

I hope that I have been able to convey here that the coming-into-being of the Living Tree Orchid Essences has been the result of a (fairly small) team effort over the past decade and more. Each one has played an important role in the creation of the line, and I am grateful for the

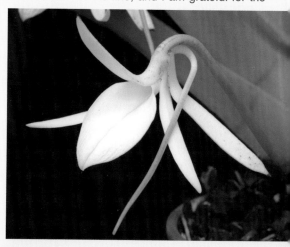

participation of each of these good friends. It has been a rare and very special collaboration, set within the broader global activities, opportunities and sharing of knowledge & insights of so many in our field. It is my hope that this book may also now in turn contribute to the process of sharing which I have found so valuable since the founding of IFER.

Pictured upper left, opposite page: *Aeranthes grandiflora* (Clear Mind). Detail opposite is of *Bulbo. phalaenopsis* (Shadow Warrior), and main photo above. Pictured to the right is a close-up of Joyous Purification, which we believe to be *Jumellea major*.

Our Essence Descriptions

We have two sections in this book for descriptions of the LTOE. Towards the end of the book are the brief descriptions we have provided for a number of years in our small brochure, which are based primarily upon the clairvoyant readings of Peter Tadd. These make mention in many instances to the essences' actions upon the above-the-body chakras. We have found over the years that many people wanted simpler descriptions, especially as these higher chakras are barely described in available literature. Nevertheless we feel there is a clear value in retaining these descriptions, and for some therapists they will provide important insights. The descriptions in that section of essences made in the past 6 years however are written either by myself and/or by Dr. Brito-Babapulle.

By contrast the pages that follow immediately contain descriptions of the essences which are generally from a rather simpler angle of approach. These are based on a mixture of feedback from therapists, of Heather's meditational insights, of Peter's understandings from his clairvoyant perspective, and also from my own experiences with the essences, both directly and from teaching in seminars over the past six years. These are also the pages with the fullest emphasis on the photos of the orchids. I have also included basic botanical information on each plant. With a few of the descriptions, the language is fairly technical, particularly Fire of Life and Furnace of Life. These essences were made by me but at the behest of Dr. Brito-Babapulle, for whom they have such importance in his work that I have given his descriptions free rein in these cases. His passion for the applied kinesiological work he has evolved, and for the orchid essences as tools within that framework of treatment, has helped bring the LTOE into areas we would not otherwise have explored, and I am grateful for his substantial input these past several years especially.

Following the Combinations pages you will find two charts, one listing which acupuncture meridians each essence resonates with, both as a primary and as a secondary resonance. The other lists which chakras resonate with each essence. Our thanks go to Linda Jeffrey for undertaking this enormous work. The chakras chart also shows (by columnar coding) which essences have essence of 24 karat Gold added as a neutral enhancer, and also who of our small group over the years made each individual LTOE. Where the person's abbreviations are in (brackets) this indicates they were involved in the making but not directly, physically involved. For example, Adrian was at home in England when he called to tell me that I needed to make an essence with the two orchids which his gifted long-term friend had seen the day before on a visit to Gigha; and so Fire of Life and Furnace of Life came to be made. This is indicated in the 3rd column as "DD(+ABB)".

Different therapists will generally find somewhat different information when approaching subtle body analysis. In the chakras listing, there were a few instances where Peter Tadd mentioned specific chakras in relation to an essence, which did not test up in Linda's very fine muscle-testing. These discrepancies are of interest I feel, and so are left as something for the reader to reflect upon. However, the spreadsheet in question in effect posed over 2,000 questions. In just over one percent of these possibilities, they arrived at divergent answers. That's a pretty high degree of correlation.

The descriptions of the combination essences and sprays are almost entirely based on the feedback we have had over the years, combined with my own experiences both directly and with others.

In brief, if a description refers much to higher chakras, that description was most likely written originally by Peter Tadd. If it refers to pulsation points, receptors and divine consciousness, then it will have been written by Adrian. If the text is a little more meandering and conversational, then most likely that's me...

Andean Fire

In the course of our many lifetimes, the trials and challenges we have faced will often have left their mark. The deeper the experience in crisis, the greater the impact on our being which can persist through time and lives. The natural courage and sense of purpose of the soul may become dimmed, unless these deep memories can be healed. Andean Fire helps one to regain the soul's natural courage, which provides the wind in the sails for pursuing our purpose.

In meditation Heather saw herself visiting scenes of overwhelming devastation, then standing at the foot of Christ on the cross. Heather touched his blood on the ground, then her heart with it, which brought about a deep shift in her; she then re-visited the scenes of devastation but was now far better able to handle herself, and be of help to others.

Phragmipedium Andean Fire is a primary cross of *Phrag. besseae* and *Phrag. lindleyanum*.

Angelic Canopy

was made a week after 9/11, and would have helped with the deep sense of despondency and deep emotional & even spiritual trauma which those terrible events engendered. We had several orchids in bloom at the time, and Heather noticed that this one, unlike the others, had not 'dimmed' in response to the trauma of spirit we all felt. When the essence was made, Heather saw a woman dressed in a chiffon gown the same colours as the orchid, carrying a bowl filled with the sweet nectar which oozes from the blooms, and as she walked around us, she sprinkled the nectar into our auras, saying "Balm for the troubled soul".

Angelic Canopy remains our most universal essence, with its wonderful sense of reassurance about the fundamental goodness of life. Applied topically it will push negative energies out of the chakras within the body. For the same reason it is very good for cleansing crystals: just place a crystal in a bowl of water, and add 3 drops of Angelic Canopy.

An extremely useful essence for anyone who is upset, anxious or feeling low. Helpful for the challenges of being a parent.

Laeliocattleya Angel Love is a warm-growing hybrid based on two genera from Central and South America. The genus Cattleya has nearly 50 species, and the genus Laelia roughly 20 species. There have been many thousands of Laeliocattleya hybrids made over the past 120 years. Most of these, like the species they derive from, are astonishingly beautiful.

Behold the Silence
has always had a brief description in our brochure which has baffled most people - showing one of the perils of working with a very fine clairvoyant! In simpler terms, what Peter was trying to say is that this orchid has an extraordinary spiritual depth, and that from that perspective, time no longer has the linear 'reality' which we generally experience. So Behold the Silence is able to bring deep healing to the soul by means we cannot readily comprehend. But imagine if we could see time like a meandering river from above; to understand that the future of the soul is as 'real' as the present and the past. Andean Fire has a kindred action, though addressing different concerns and aspects.

Primarily what one experiences when taking this essence is simply a beautiful quality of inner silence. This is quite different from the silent stillness of Secret Wisdom, as this silence has a sense of flow and gentle, deep movement. The consciousness of this orchid is highly evolved, and in seminar it is one of the last essences we experience. We generally need to acclimatise to the very high and refined energy it wishes to share with us.

Comparetia macroplectron is a specie native to the cloud forests of Colombia.

Being in Time
A little devic lady in pantaloons said to Heather when we had just finished making the mother tincture, "This one's really special", pointing at the orchid. And over time we have come to see that this is one of our most useful essences for modern living. On the one hand it provides remarkable help in adjusting to the local time zone after long distance flights. On the other hand, it helps people whose body-clocks have become askew to re-align with the cycles of nature. Electromagnetic radiation of all the sorts we are bombarded with will tend to wreak havoc with our body's natural rhythms, so this is one of the essences which is able to help counteract that.

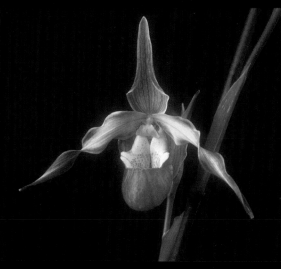

Being in Time is also very helpful for those who feel they have too much to do, and too little time in which to do it. The essence will bring a more graceful sense to the flow of time in one's day. So if you have to suddenly get ready for a flight abroad, take it while packing, and when you land, to make the entire journey far easier.

Phragmipedium Ainsworthii is one of the earliest hybrids created in this genus, dating back to 1879. It is a cross of *Phrag. longifolium var. roezlii* and *Phragmipedium Sedenii*.

Being in Grace is one of the range

which has both remedial & enhancer aspects. Heather's meditational experience describes the enhancer quality very clearly: she saw herself sitting on a throne, with robes the beautiful purple colour of the orchid. All was calm and regal, and lovely.

However, if a person is sitting on left-over old emotions, which have been brushed under the carpet of the psyche, then the first time that person takes the drops, they are likely to find that the carpet is lfted as it were, so that they become consciously aware of the old feelings they had been hiding within. This moment of awareness can be uncomfortable, but the very simple solution is to take the drops a second time, just a few minutes after the first drops. This will nearly always bring instant relief, as the emotions are cleansed from the psyche and aura.

In effect the orchid wants you to first become aware of the emotions it is about to clear away. Only then is the next step of the healing process possible. This two-step process arises in fewer than one person in ten who try the essence. Most people will only experience the lovely enhancer aspect of Being in Grace, but where the remedial quality is needed, it is a powerful tool.

Ascocenda Princess Mikasa is a Vandaceous hybrid which likes warmth and plenty of light.

Boundless Peace is one of the most yin essences in the line, and is likely to have

an impact on the dream state. Heather and I had finished the making of the essence late one evening, and I found when I went to bed that night, I seemed to dream all night long. There are reasons we don't sell the mother tincture! At stock strength this is a very good essence for helping one to unwind at the end of a stressful day, and it is one of the components of both

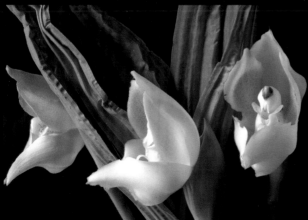

Gentle Geisha and Gentle Sleep, as well as Sleep of Peace. Men may especially benefit if they need feeding of the yin aspect to help balance their yang energy.

Anguloa virginalis is a specie native to the cool cloud forests of the mountains of Peru. It is a plant with very large leaves, which likes frequent watering.

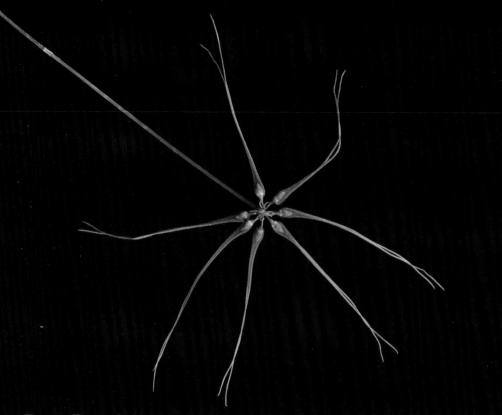

Base Regulator is a very powerful essence with several layers of activity. There is a profound effect on the pelvic centres as well as on the crown chakra. It establishes a countercurrent in the pelvis, reining in excess sexual energies. Base Regulator also has a powerful effect on the liver in reducing heat in the organ.

This essence is very useful if one's sexual drive is too powerful. The effect on one person was a strong and clear damping-down of his excessive sexual drive to a healthy level, one which was no longer tormenting. He described the reduction in libido as dramatic, painless and gratefully experienced. For one woman there was an immediate cessation of her period and the associated painful symptoms. There is a shift of energy from the pelvic region to higher centres, experienced as a rapid expansion of consciousness radiating out (mainly 'sideways') from the head in all directions, just as the blooms themselves are seen facing every direction.

This physical aspect of the orchid is worth noting and reflecting on. Whereas Necklace of Beauty and Pushing Back the Night (whose orchids are related to this one) present their multiple blooms in roughly a 120 degree spread, Bulbophyllum gracillimum presents its multiple blooms facing 360 degrees. The essence was made over a 16 hour period, during most of which time the orchid looked much as it appears in the photo above, with the sexual parts of the blooms not yet revealed. This is the key contrast with Core Release, which was made with the fully-open blooms entirely.

With Base Regulator, as excess yang sexual energy is reined in, one experiences a beautiful and deep delicacy in relation to one's sexuaity. At the same time there is a strengthening of one's higher spiritual connection within the framework of the greatly expanded consciousness.

Core Release

This orchid is one of the few in our range which gave rise to two essences, related yet quite distinct in their actions.

Whereas Base Regulator (opposite page) was made when the sexual parts of the blooms (the white & yellow elements seen in the photos) were still concealed within the dark red forms of the petals, Core Release was made later in the bloom cycle, with the blooms fully developed as seen in the photo here. (The blooms of *Bulbophyllum gracillimum* last approximately 3 to 4 days.)

The energetic differences are substantial. As with Base Regulator, Core Release has a major impact on the pulsation points of the pelvic region, but without the damping impact on the libido. Core Release enhances the sexual centre's sensitivity, and at the same time brings an element of protection to the entire pelvic area. This is a highly unusual feature of this essence, which we have not encountered with any other essence. Core Release also brings an impetus to get on with things one needs to do, through its action on both the 3rd chakra and the Ajana centre. Moreover one's intuitive abilities are heightened. As it is a very new essence, our understanding of it will be developing further in the months ahead; this information will be shared on our website. As one can see, our work with the LTOE is an on-going process of exploration and research. *(We have left the chakra and meridian chart information blank at this stage; later editions will complete these. However it is already clear that this is a major essence.)*

Bulbophyllum gracillimum is an epiphyte found in humid lowland forests in Thailand, Myanmar, Malaysia and the Solomon Islands. It was first described botanically in 1897.

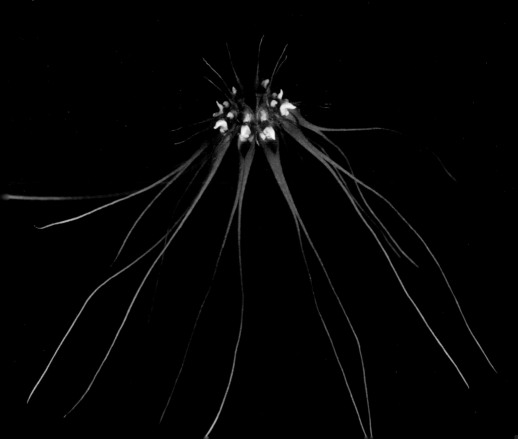

Celestial Siren is one of our most recently-made essences, capturing Adrian's attention when he came to Gigha in November 2009 to teach a kinesiology workshop. I had only recently brought this orchid back from a trip to Germany.

The genus Dendrobium is one of the two largest in the family orchidaceae with over 1,200 species, all found in SE Asia. Most of them have long pseudobulbs which grow upwards from the branch of a tree, but in this section they hang down. With Dendrobium lawesii, which is a native of Papua New Guinea, the blooms also grow facing down, but with a thin tube called the nectary growing back up. There is considerable colour varietion in this specie, from oranges to reds to pinks.

The experience in meditation mirrors this posture, with one's head bent forward, and then a movement of energy back up through the face and then through the rear top of the head. And then once this inner and outer posture has shifted, stillness. This is a stillness so deep and rich, one can stay within it for hours, maybe even days.

The day after the essence was made I took a nap in the afternoon, and dreamt of seeing a monk in robes, sitting beside a calm lake in meditation, with the golden light of the sun streaming down on him and the lake. For Adrian and myself, this image conveys the essence of Celestial Siren's teaching.

Carnival helps to remind us that a part of our spiritual journey is to learn to live in harmony and joy with our body and our senses, and to be able to enjoy the sensual side of life. The Puritan repression of the body created an artificial division between Spirit and Body; Carnival helps bring healing to that division, to enable the healthy dance of joy of the incarnate spirit. This essence helps awaken the sensual life of the skin especially, the exquisite surface of our being.

Very good for incorporating in a beauty or skin cream. Combines with Laughing Butterflies to make the combination Party Time!

I was sold the orchid as a specimen of *Laelia crispa*, but as can often happen in the orchid world, the commercial seller was wrong. So at this time all we can say about the beautiful orchid which produced Carnival is that it is an unidentified Laeliocattleya hybrid.

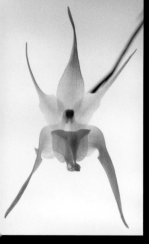

Clear Mind

Clear Mind was made during a full moon on a clear, still and cold night, with a very clear piece of aquamarine in the bowl of water. This orchid is active at night, when it gives off a fragrance like butterscotch, this fragrance not being there in the day. A very good essence for helping to calm the mind when you need to reflect on things, or when studying. One customer used it to keep calm when engaged in Formula One racing. Very much an essence for the mental body, as seen by it acting primarily on the Ajana Centra, Bahui point and the crown chakra.

Aeranthes grandiflora is a specie native to Madagascar.

Core of Being

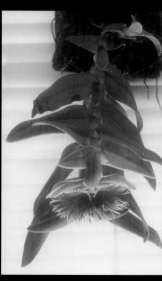

Core of Being is a very unusual orchid, and its energy is very calming yet also strengthening. Before we had started exploring the orchids, Peter Tadd said to me that he didn't think any flower essence could reach the level of the Causal body. Yet that is where Peter saw his essence go directly, thereby helping the alignment of all the chakras indirectly. Core of Being has an inward movement. For example, when added to our combination Double Espresso it creates another combination we call Vital Lift. In effect it contains' that expansive yang energy. Core of Being is suitable for anyone feeling tired or pressed by the demands of the day, and may be taken at any time of the day or night.

Nanodes medusae is a native of the cloud forests of Ecuador.

Clearing the Way / Self Belief

Clearing the Way / Self Belief is very good for anyone who suffers from a lack of self-confidence, who doesn't believe that they have the inner resources to achieve what they would wish to do. This is a gently yang essence, which we have seen be of great help to many people over the years. The impact is fairly noticeable when the drops are taken, and so it is often the essence I will give to a sceptical visitor who doubts essences can have any real effect.

Phragmipedium Don Wimbur is a second generation besseae hybrid, in other words, *Phrag. besseae* is one of the parents in both generations. And it is via *Phrag. besseae* that the strong yang quality comes through in Clearing the Way / Self Belief. *Phrag. longifolium* was crossed with *Phrag. besseae* to produce *Phrag. Eric Young*, which was in turn crossed with *Phrag. besseae* to produce *Phrag. Don Wimbur.*

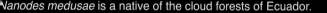

Direct Vision was made with the same orchid which produced New Vitality, but six months earlier. Simply the orientation of the two blooms led to the two essences having very different qualities. With Direct Vision the two blooms were facing the same direction, just as you see here.

Heather & Natalie & I all had very powerful experiences of the 3rd eye when we had sipped the mother tincture, though this effect is eased by the dilution down to stock strength (which is how all of the LTOE are sold). Heather had a new guide who entered the proceedings with this essence: a Native American. He had a serious demeanour, and regarded this essence as a useful tool for vision quests. It can also be used for awakening the brow chakra. This is not an essence to be used lightly, but treated with a certain respect.

Paphipedilum liemianum is native to the limestone hills of northern Sumatra. It is a sequential bloomer, and a single spike can keep producing blooms for over 18 months, with each bloom lasting roughly 6 weeks. The green staminode cap at the centre of the bloom conceals the principal sexual parts of the orchid.

Crown of Consciousness

It took Peter several months to do his 'reading' of this essence, and when I asked him why, he said that he had felt intimidated by the prospect. Why? "Because its like being asked to do a reading of the Dalai Lama". For Peter it was clear that this orchid embodied very sacred energies, that approaching it was to come into the presence of highly evolved being. "When this orchid comes into bloom, the whole Earth knows it" he said.

This orchid's name *Masdevallia regina* means it is the Queen of the genus, and rightly so in my view. An epiphytic specie native to the cool cloud forests of Peru, it is a glory to behold when in flower. The bloom can be up to 14" from tip to tip, with remarkable patterns and colouring. There have been over 600 species of Masdevallia found so far.

One of our customers wrote the following to us last year: "I have had 2 amazing meditation experiences, one in Thailand and one back here, while taking it. I would say that the name is very apt. What I felt and saw was out of human consiousness, out of the awareness. It was beyond anything I have ever experienced and I feel so blessed that it happened."

These two essences and their combination act upon the Ming men (translation - gate of destiny). They relate strongly to the masculine and feminine within us all.

The Ming men is located in the low back, inbetween the second and third lumbar vertebra. In Chinese medicine it is called the Gate of Destiny because it holds all of our potential for life. The Ming men contains the initial spark of life that expands out to give power to the organs, channels and substances of the body.

The Ming men is the union of the masculine and feminine energies. When in harmony they unite to harness the power and fire of the kundalini energy, allowing it to rise up the spine and connect to the universal energy. This fire is the 'fuel' for the evolution process.

If the fire of the Ming men dwindles or is extinguished, then there is separation between the male and female (between yin and yang). This leads to illness, disease and a limited belief system in the individual.

Furnace of Life

This is the female counterpart of this pair of essences (orchid resembles the female genitalia), and allows one to see situations and life decisions with truth and clarity. The essence brings you into an inner sanctuary of peace, in close contact with the divine, a womb-like sensation with a deep sense of being nurtured.

Fire of Life

This is the male counterpart (the form of the bloom suggests the male genitalia) this breathes life into the dwindling flames of the Ming Men and strengthens personal will, to make choices in line with the divine energy, setting them on the path to their true destiny. Please note: both of these essences contain essence of 24 karat Gold.

Spirit of Life is the combination of these two essences.

Physically, this essence realigns the vertebral system, emotionally it gives one a sense of clarity (knowing). Spiritually it strengthens the resolve and reveals the purpose of the spiritual journey. Energetically it raises the vitality of the pelvic energy centres.

Masdevallia ignea (on the right) is found growing terrestrially on the cloud-forest floor in Colombia at 3,000 meters.

Masdevallia veitchiana (top) grows terrestrially or lithophytically in full sun at 2,300 to 3,900 meters in the mountains of Peru.

Golden Radiance

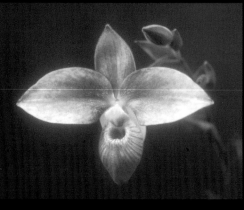

Golden Radiance was the first essence Heather and I made together, and the innate approach of deep respect which Heather brought to the process was wonderful to witness and participate in. Golden Radiance helps us to connect with the radiance of our inner heart, and shifts us away from negativity.

Though Unveiling Affection (*Phrag. Hanne Popow*) is one of the parents of this hybrid, its action is very different. Still relating to the heart, this essence helps us to tap the deep well-springs of the heart, enabling an overall shift in our outlook, to see, sense and contribute to the goodness and the joy of our relationships. Like an air freshener for the spirits, Golden Radiance will brighten your day.

Phragmipedium Saint Ouen is a cross of *Phrag. Hanne Popow* and *Phragmipedium besseae*. It was registered by the Eric Young Orchid Foundation on the island of Jersey in 1996.

Guardian of the Inner Journey

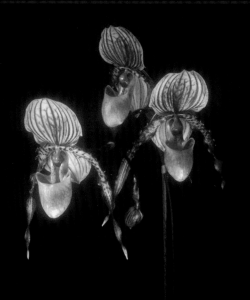

Guardian of the Inner Journey Several of the Paphiopedilum essences are fairly serious, none more so than this one. There is a time and place for all things, and sometimes it is appropriate for us to take the question of our spiritual path more seriously. Have we perhaps been neglecting it? For some people, meditating with this essence can be quite intense, and may leave one feeling ungrounded. We therefore always recommend that anyone wishing to work with Guardian of the Inner Journey also have on hand Walking to the Earth's Rhythm - which just happened to be the next essence that Heather and I made.

My dots were very clear that these two essences are a kind of 'working' pair. Take Guardian of the Inner Journey at the start of one's meditation, and Walking to the Earth's Rhythm at the end. This is somewhat akin to taking off in a plane, and then landing it - the latter skill is rather important.

Paphiopedilum Helvetia is a primary cross of *Paph. chamberlainianum* with *Paph. philippinense.*

Healing the Higher Heart

was the first essence which Adrian and I made together, just prior to Shadow Warrior. Adrian was transfixed by this orchid the moment he set foot in the greenhouse. He immediately knew that this would provide an essence for helping the "higher heart chakra", which is located just above the heart chakra itself. One function of the higher heart chakra is to help maintain the health of the heart chakra; but if the higher heart chakra becomes unhealthy, then the entire heart chakra system gets stuck in an unhealthy pattern.

Often the first time someone takes this essence, they will feel a brief wave of grief washing through and out of their heart, as the higher heart chakra now begins once more to do its work. Healing the Higher Heart (or HHH for short) differs from Spirit of the Higher Heart in having the addition of 5 drops of 24 karat Gold essence added to the bottle. Start with HHH, and follow up with Spirit of the Higher Heart.

See Spirit of the Higher Heart for further botanical notes regarding *Vascostylis Roll on Red*.

Hara to Heart helps with the healthy flow of energies between and through our chakras. If there is a disconnection between the heart and the second (sexual) chakra, then all sorts of troubles arise in our life. Hara to Heart helps these two and the 3rd chakra (seat of will and action) engage in a harmonious flow, from the 2nd up through the 3rd and into the heart chakra. Unless we have this grounding our spiritual path will be beset with obstacles of our own creation.

Peter saw that once the first trio of chakras were in a healthy flow, then the essence moves to another higher trio. Linda Jeffrey in her muscle-testing confirmed what Peter had seen several years before, of the next trio being the 8th, 9th and 10th chakras. An interesting exercise therefore is to sit while taking this essence, and sense its action moving up through the chakras; see where it takes you. An important essence for helping the foundation of our spiritual path.

Bulbophyllum lobbii is widespread in SE Asia from northeastern India to the Philippines. It has a lovely fragrance which would make a good perfume. It's lip easily bobbles back & forth if there is a breeze. There are at least several dozen varieties of this epiphytic specie

Internal Cleansing was the only orchid we have made an essence with where the impulse was intellectual curiousity. I came upon it in bloom at an orchid show, and while some orchids have a lovely fragrance (but most have very little or none) this one has a different pollination strategy: it stinks like dung, which attracts blowflies. In retrospect it seems utterly obvious that it should act on the large intestine especially. But at the time I had a conceptual block.

Both Heather and Peter saw the same devic fellow, a tall lanky being with long fingers, whom Heather saw leaning over a pile of entrails, and was picking through it. "Not very nice!" said Heather, to which he replied, "Maybe so, but someone has to do it..."

Internal Cleansing helps with the health of the digestive system from the liver down through the large intestine. It also has higher purposes, but its energetic nature is distinct enough that it asked to be wrapped in foil if it was to be stored next to the other orchid essences.

Bulbophyllum echinolabium is a specie native to Sulawesi, with the largest single bloom in the genus, sometimes measuring 15" (38cm) from tip to tip. Often in bloom in our greenhouse, it makes its presence known as soon as you enter.

Heart of Light was made with the same hybrid which
produced Messenger of the Heart, although it was a different specimen. That one type of hybrid could produce two very different essences was a very significant part of our learning curve.

Somehow the two spikes had brought forth blooms which were almost facing each other. Natalie's involvement in the making helped bring through higher chakra activity. Heart of Light helps to remove blockages from the heart chakra, and can be a good follow-up to Messenger of the Heart. Without fanfare it helps one to access the heart's higher knowledge.

Phragmipedium Grouville is a cross of *Phragmipedium Hanne Popow* & *Phrag. Eric Young*. The deep red *Phrag. besseae* is a 'grandparent' on both sides. *Phrag. Grouville* was registered by the Eric Young Orchid Foundation on the island of Jersey in 1996.

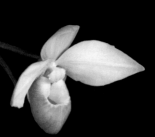

Just Me

Just Me This orchid grabbed Natalie's attention the moment she saw it - always a good sign. It spoke to her at levels beyond conscious awareness, of how it could help her and others of unusual character.

If we don't readily fit the 'normal' parameters and expectations of society, we are likely to feel a degree of alone-ness. Emotionally there are times when this status within the community is hard to take. Just Me helps one to be accepting of who one is, and to be comfortable with not being with the 'in crowd'. In any case, who wants to be run-of-the-mill?

Cochlioda noezliana is a native of the cloud forests of northern Peru, where it grows epiphytically & sometimes lithopytically at elevations of 2,000 to 3,500 meters.

Joyous Purification

Joyous Purification told Peter that the entire form of the plant was significant. Note how the nearly pure white blooms arise from the base of the plant, which correlates to the purifying action of the essence on the 1st & 2nd chakras. And the whole plant seems to be dancing, as seen in the photo, which suggests the joy which the name of the essence refers to, as well as the movement of energies it facilitates. Acts as well on the Dan Tien (perineal point). This is one of the LTOE which helps in the psychological healing process for those who have experienced sexual abuse. By releasing old grief and emotional residue from the root chakra, it helps one to retrieve the connection with one's deeper purpose in life. Joyous Purification is a very good adjunct to the action of Sacral Regulator.

Jumellea major is from northern Madagascar and is found in lowland forest up to 1,500 metres. There are roughly 60 species of Jumellea, all found in Madagascar , the Comoro Islands, Mascarene Islands, and two species are found on mainland Africa.

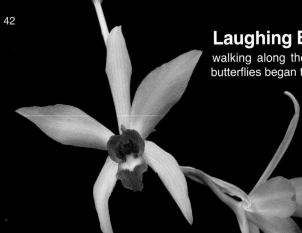

Laughing Butterflies
Heather saw herself walking along the bed of a stream, when suddenly butterflies began to come out of her mouth, larger and larger butterflies the colours of this orchid. When we meditated we were quite serious about what we were doing. So how does the psyche convey humour in symbolic terms to the consciously serious mind? This was a perfect image. Laughing Butterflies helps us to lighten up and enjoy the dance of life. The swirling inner and outer movement of yin and yang should be enjoyed and celebrated!

Laelia anceps is an epiphyte native to Mexico and Guatemala. Flowering in winter, its spike can be up to a meter long.

Knight's Cloak
was made by Dominic and Heather after our friend Rose Titchiner had drawn Dominic's attention to the orchid after a visit to the Living Tree. The leaf shields the bloom, which holds deep within its dark purple form a tiny golden sphere, almost too small to see by the naked eye.

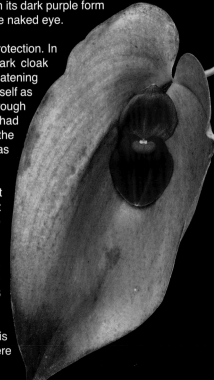

This is one of our principal essences for psychic protection. In meditation Dominic saw himself wrapped in a dark cloak which kept him safe by not being seen by the threatening black flames he was walking past. Heather saw herself as a musketeer, jumping on a horse and galloping through the night, unseen thanks to the dark cloak she had wrapped around herself. When we called Peter on the phone, his first comment about the new essence was "there's something very 'cloaky' about it..."

Later, Peter told me to make a note of the fact that it stengthened and protected the back of the Throat Chakra specifically. I told him I didn't think we needed to make the information that specific, but he insisted. "Don, the back of the throat chakra is the first area hit in a psychic attack. And it is more vulnerable in women than in men. You need to note this down." Knight's Cloak is of course one of the 3 components of Soul Shield.

Pleurothallis gargantua is a native of Ecuador and is found in the mountains in the cool cloud forests. There are well over 600 species of Pleurothallis.

Liberation / Deception

Perhaps we should have come up with a different name for this essence, because although accurately descriptive, the name makes this a very difficult essence to recommend to someone! Nobody wants to believe that they deceive themselves, yet that is a part of the human condition... Although we know how to think, we are not inherently *good* at thinking. We are inclined to give absolute value to ideas and beliefs, when such absolute value distorts any critical thinking relating to that idea or belief.

In his reading of this essence, Peter had the orchid in bloom in front of him, which presented a puzzling image to him: that of a white stone buddha wearing a Rastefarian hat. Then he saw Che Guevara, and one or two other 'revolutionaries'. Finally Peter said, "Ah, this orchid is about the way we deceive ourselves in the name of liberation." And the orchid said to him, "Now you've got it!". In other words, we find it difficult to think clearly if we have given extraordinarily high value to an idea or belief. Ideas should be able to be discussed and examined, but if we think we have found "The One True Path" then all other related thinking becomes distorted. Liberation / Deception helps us to refine the self-reflective aspect of our mental process.

I once found that a woman muscle-tested very strongly for this essence, which had surprised me, until I learnt that organic food was for her the most important thing in her life. Each day life was made difficult for anyone close to her by her insistence on every effort being made to find the organic food she demanded. It was far beyond any appropriate level of importance. I then discovered that it can be very difficult, and even impossible to try to explain to someone why you think they need this essence. In her view I was simply WRONG and she was deeply offended. My recommendation therefore is simply to give the essence to a person if in your view they need it. Let the essence do its work, and do not attempt too much explanation!

When a person is feeling low, a negative feedback loop is created between thoughts and feelings. This essence will help break that loop, and provide one with a clearer perspective on one's deeply-held beliefs.

The Oxford philosopher F.H. Bradley once wrote* "...if we are to think, we should sometimes try to think properly." I believe that this orchid would wish to agree.

Paphiopedilum gratixianum is a specie native to Vietnam and Laos, where it grows on the forest floor, with its roots spread under the leaf litter.

* In the 1893 Introduction to *Appearance & Reality*

Light of My Eye
This essence was made by Heather and me, with our friends David Carson & his daughter Greta having helped in the lead up to the making when they were in Milland on a visit. Heather saw herself in a subterranean chamber when we meditated on this essence; she then followed a light which she could see in a tunnel. She felt the essence gave her more strength and perseverance to carry on the journey up the tunnel towards the light.

Adrian has done further research on the qualities of this essence, and the description that follows here is his.

The activity of the essence is to enhance the visual cortex and open the third eye and Ajana point, to bring one to see light above light (Divine light). This essence can have very distinct physical effects stemming from the way in which it brings etheric light into the eyeballs themselves.

This essence immediately brings increased clarity with the eye drawn to physical details. It also helps one to see connections and disconnections in the aura in a manner similar to Shadow Warrior, but with much more clarity of detail. There is also a sense of knowledge stemming from the higher chakras, mainly from the 14th chakra.

Paphiopedilum Memoria Richard Ong is a cross of *Paph. Michael Koopowitz* and *Paph. lowii*, which was registered by Jason Ong of Brooklyn, New York in 2001.

Mercutio
This essence is especially helpful for children who are either lacking self-confidence at school, or who are subject to verbal threats and verbal bullying, or worse. In these situations, the lung meridian 'freezes up' from the flight vs. fight reflex mingled with fear. The effect of this circumstance on the playground at school can be that the child's verbal development is inhibited. Mercutio helps the lungs to un-freeze, so the throat chakra is then able to play its role.

Recently in working with Adrian, we found that this was one of ten essences in the range that wanted to have essence of 24 karat Gold added to it as an enhancer.

Pleurothallis restrepioides is a specie found growing epiphytically and terrestrially in the cloud forests of Colombia, Ecuador and Peru. It was described by the great botanist John Lindley in 1836, the same year he began to lecture at the Chelsea Physic Garden in London.

Life Direction (Lanata)

There are close to 50 species in this genus from the cloud forests of South America, and we have made essences with just two of them so far. There is so much yet to explore!

The night after first seeing this orchid in the greenhouse, Natalie dreamt she was walking through the desert, not knowing where she should go, which direction to take. She turned around, and there just in front of her face was this orchid 'looking' at her, though it was in the dream far larger than in real life. Natalie told me of her dream the next day, and it was quite clear to me both what the dream was saying, and also that we needed to make an essence with the orchid.

Sure enough, the orchid helps one with finding one's direction in life. The form of the bloom is of interest: it looks rather like a bow and arrow. If you picture drawing an arrow back in a bow in order to take aim, this image tells you a great deal about the essence. It is not about the shooting of the arrow, it is that moment of the pulling back in towards one, the taking aim. Similarly on a physical level it helps those who are highly sensitive, to better cope with the sensory overload of big urban environments. It helps the nerves to pull back from the constant stimulus a city offers. One therapist living in London's East End said this essence was a "life-saver" for him.

Scaphosepalum swertifolium is an epiphyte found between 750 and 2300 meters up in the cloud forests of Colombia and Ecuador. The flower spike will produce several or many blooms in succession. The blooms are roughly 2 inches wide, so the bloom above is larger than lifesize.

Messenger of the Heart

was made just seven months after Unveiling Affection. Peter saw a messenger on a white horse galloping along in my heart chakra when I took the drops on his next visit to The Living Tree. One customer took the essence and that evening she finally had a long talk with her boyfriend, in which she was able to speak about things she had been sitting on for many months. This is very much an essence to help you give voice to your heartfelt feelings.

Phragmipedium Grouville is a second generation hybrid, a cross of *Phrag. Hanne Popow* and *Phrag. Eric Young*. The deep red *Phrag. besseae* is a 'grandparent' on both sides. Clearly the discovery in 1981 of *Phragmipedium besseae* has led to a wonderful explosion of hybridizing activity. *Phrag. Grouville* was registered by the Eric Young Orchid Foundation on the island of Jersey in 1996.

45

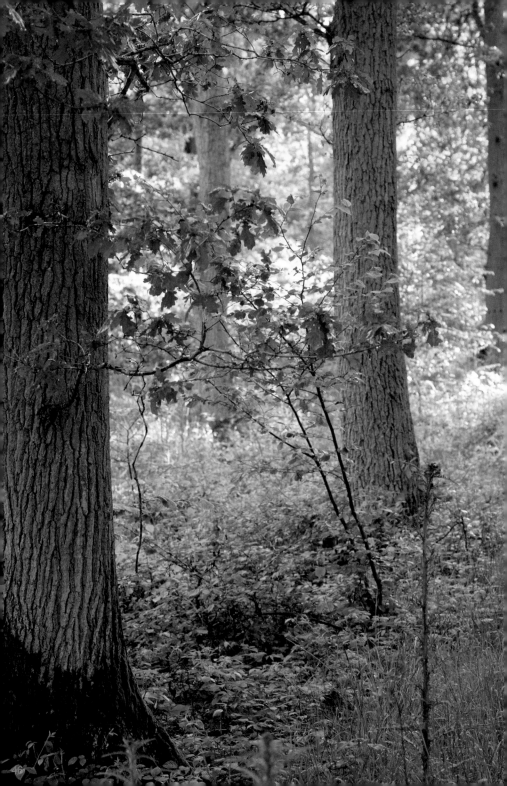

Hatch Copse & the Narnia Sphagnum Moss

How important are the few remaining magical places in the world... and how easily are they lost. There was one such wonderful woodland a mile from our old premises in the Milland valley, a 10 acre wood called Hatch Copse. Planted as an oak woodland over a century before, it was regarded by locals as somehow special. But to anyone outside of Milland it was simply invisible, one of those places that people simply rarely visit. I have fond memories of playing Pooh Sticks with Arthur Bailey in the little brook shown below, where Natalie is sitting. This was a woodland favoured by nature spirits for whom it was a sanctuary, a place in our world where they could be in their element, in a secluded woodland which was largely ignored by humanity.

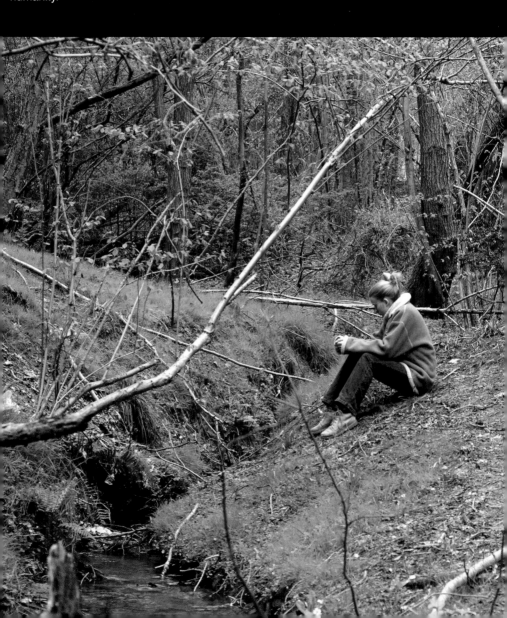

One day Heather, Natalie, Peter and I went for a walk in Hatch Copse, and in the course of exploring in various parts of the wood, Natalie came upon a large boggy area covered in the most vibrant sphagnum moss any of us had ever seen. Peter commented that it would be great to make an essence with it, which Natalie and I did a few days later. We simply placed a bowl of water on top of the bed of moss (as you see below), and left it for several hours. This moss was so vibrant, we both felt there was simply no need to pick any of it to place some in the bowl: the energy of the moss would be filling the bowl without that being done. And we wished to disturb the moss as little as possible. After several hours we poured an equal measure of brandy to the water, and poured the mother tincture into the large bottles we had brought for the purpose.

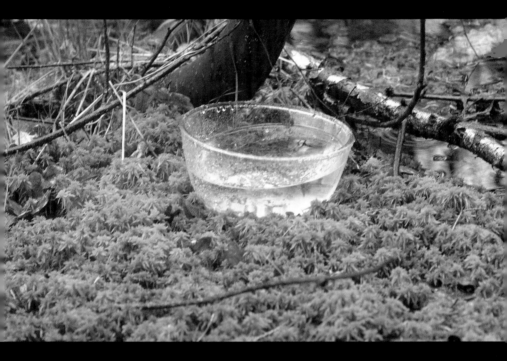

The full story of this woodland, and the making of this essence, is told on our website. And there is much to tell. Both for SSK and for Peter the wood was a favourite place to visit when they would come to see us at the Living Tree, as both were able to see many nature spirits there. Even those of us without clairvoyant abilities could feel the extraordinary magic of the place. Peter took to calling it "Narnia", and hence when the essence was made it we called it the Narnia Sphagnum Moss.

A few years later, authorized tree-felling took place with no regard for the nature of the wood, and much of its special magic was lost. This is the same story that has been repeated over many centuries across the whole of Europe and elsewhere. The story line of the new film "Avatar", and of "Fern Gully" before it, sadly are based in reality. We have to learn a new

Positive Outcome
helps us to maintain a positive frame of mind. I have often said that I could make a good case for this being the most important essence in our range, for the simple reason that this essence addresses an issue which affects our lives, day by day, minute by minute, and year by year. If we expect the day to be miserable, guess what we will almost always experience on that day? Having a positive attitude is not about wearing rose-tinted glasses; it is about seeing the possibilities that are always present. Moreover, in the current "global financial crisis" it is all too easy to succumb to the dark fog which has descended on the national psyche, which has largely been created by the media. Positive Outcome encourages us to be positive, and not to give in to our fears. With a positive frame of mind, all challenges become easier to resolve, and new opportunities will present themselves.

Scaphosepalum gibberosum is native to the cloud forests of Colombia and Ecuador. It has the largest bloom of this genus of roughly 45 species, and a single flower spike can be in bloom for up to five years.

Protective Presence
is an extraordinary and bizarre-looking orchid from Papua New Guinea and neighbouring islands. I believe that the warriors of PNG must have taken their style of body painting from this orchid, which in the past would have been fairly common on the branches of trees there.

The blooms are also reminiscent of the "wrathful deities" of Tibetan Buddhism, which are seen in their paintings; these figures are protectors of those on their spiritual path. And so it is with this orchid, as it provides a kind of 'bodyguard' on the energetic level. It was several years into our making of essences before my dots indicated it was appropriate for us to make an essence with *Dendrobium spectabile*. Perhaps it simply wanted to be approached with a good measure of respect. A key element of our Soul Shield combination.

Dendrobium spectabile grows epiphytically and sometimes lithophytically in lowland forests of Papua New Guinea, the Solomon Islands, Vanuatu and Bougainville Island.

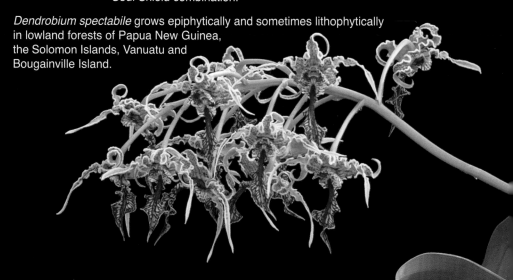

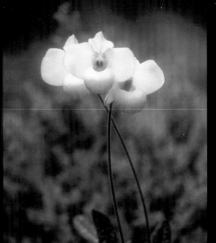

Purity of Heart would be helpful for

anyone who rushes around in their life, busy with too many tasks. Akin to Walking to the Earth's Rhythm is some ways, in that this essence invites us to experience a different rhythm and pace in our day. However this invitation sounds in our heart. Especially good for parents, to help them to be with their children, to give them the time and the patience that they need for their nurture. If we can create unhurried time for our children, they will feel valued and loved, and our hearts will open.

Paphiopedilum Armeni White is a primary hybrid, a cross of *Paph. armeniacum* and *Paph. delenatii which was registered in 1987.*

Pushing Back the Night is one of the major essences in the line. It is hard to

know where to begin... This essence is a major essence for our higher alignment, that is, to keep our entire etheric field in health. An example: when the US began to bomb Baghdad on March 19th 2003, that evening I became terribly dizzy, almost unable to stand. This persisted the following day, so I called Peter, who said my higher chakras had been "knocked sideways" by the bombing, and I needed to take Pushing Back the Night. The dizziness stopped immediately upon my taking the drops. This is one illustration of the way in which this essence can help us to not lose our own spiritual alignment, even if the world around us is behaving in a crazy manner. We are not able to be effective help, if we lose our inner equilibrium.

Heather saw herself involved in various scenarios during our meditation, each describing a mastery of the four parts of our life: physical, emotional, mental and spiritual. Once this foundation is in place, Pushing Back the Night helps to build a golden temple in the higher chakras. It also strengthens the belt of the 3rd chakra, and the Ajana centre. Peter saw this essence working at both personal and global levels, to help give us further strength to handle any dark times humanity may bring upon itself in the years ahead.

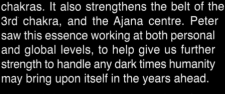

Though this essence is in a number of our combinations, we highly recommend giving it time in meditation on its own, so that you may feel its gifts directly.

Bulbophyllum Elizabeth Ann 'Buckleberry' is a primary cross of *Bulbophyllum longissimum* and *Bulbophyllum rothschildianum.*

Releasing Karmic Patterns

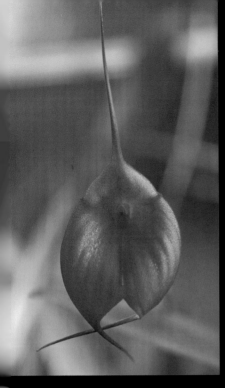

We had an unusual experience in the making of this essence. A few days after we had made it, was describing it to SSK in Alaska over the phone "Oh, the mother tincture needs to be put under the orchid again," she said. SSK simply heard this from the devic realm as we were talking. Heather and were taken aback, as we had never heard of such a procedure, but we did as she said, and she was spot on. I held a little bit back so Peter could compare the two, and it was clear that the second round of the essence under the bloom had added substantially to its qualities.

Peter's reading of the essence gave rise to lengthy discussions about the 8th chakra, and its tendency to retain specific 'heavy' (or Plutonic) patterns from past lives. The essence does not release karma - no essence can do that I believe - but it helps dissolve the karmic patterns held just above the region of the crown chakra.

Masdevallia Flying Colours is a stunning hybrid. The genus Masdevallia has over 600 species mainly found in the cloud forests of South America.

Redemption Dream

Redemption Dream has a pronounced impact on the dream state, and much of its action is effected within the theatre of our dreams as well. Deeply hidden feelings of guilt or shame, sometimes stretching back in to past lives, are likely to surface and be resolved in a non-threatening way by taking Redemption Dream over a week to 10 days. This helps clear blockages to the higher heart centre as well, since emotions like shame and guilt suppress its activity. It is also one of the essences which invokes a deep and serene calm when used in meditation, and is able to bring a deeper & fuller awareness of the soul's journey.

The orchid had come into bloom with twin flower spikes early in the winter. Then just as these two blooms faded, two more spikes developed. This was highly unusual growth, and was like a loud knock on the door from the devic realm.

Both a remedy as well as an enhancer, it is suitable for virtually everyone.

Paphiopedilum spicerianum is found on limestone hills in northeastern India and northwest Myanmar.

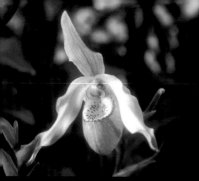

Renewing Life When this orchid came into bloom, I would sit for half an hour in the greenhouse and simply gaze at it, it was so simply beautiful and quiet. In my imagination the bloom was like a little monk in meditation, surrounded by stillness.

The action of this essence requires some explanation, and I am grateful to Peter for his description. He saw it clearing ancient negative energy patterns from the root chakra. This is the chakra which governs the patterns of cellular growth, so clearing negative energies from it has significant implications, which we are not permitted to write about. The action on the higher chakras (above the body) augments this action considerably. Nevertheless, this is a very subtle essence, very quiet and yet gently touching the heart.

Phragmipedium Carol Kanzer is a primary hybrid, a cross of *Phragmipedium pearcei* and *Phragmipedium schlimii*. The genus Phragmipedium is found in Central & South America.

Rising to the Call of Beauty is arguably one of the most important essences

in the line. When Peter did his reading of the essence, a being appeared to him above the photo of the orchid, and explained that humanity is at a crucial crossroads in its history at the moment. We have a choice of either working in harmony with the deep impulse of the evolving beauty of form which is inherent in Nature, or we can pursue the route of genetic manipulation, of both plants and animals, and even ourselves. Its power is hugely seductive. But that will move us away from natural beauty, and into realms of unintended and bizarre forms.

Those of us working with flower essences need to articulate a different vision of our planet's future, a vision based on our working in harmony with the gifts & the beauty of Nature. This hybrid is a very good example of humans working in harmony with nature. Two species were simply crossed to create an orchid of exquisite form.

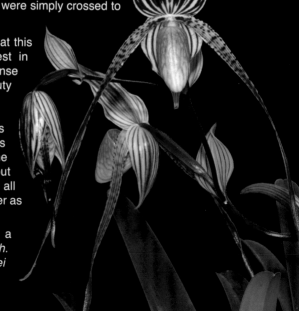

Several of our customers found that this essence created a strong interest in Feng Shui, as well as bringing a sense of joy. Rising to the Call of Beauty also helps to relax the shoulders.

One of the finest Paph. hybridizers in the USA, Jerry Fischer of Orchids Limited, commented to me that the striking and unusual thing about *Paphiopedilum Lady Isabel* is that all the hybrids that result from using her as a parent are themselves beautiful.

Paphiopedilum Lady Isabel is a primary hybrid, a cross of *Paph. rothschildianum* and *Paph. stonei* which was first registered in 1897.

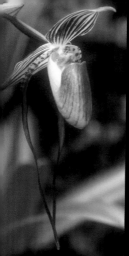

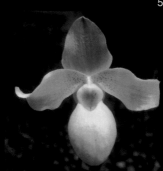

Serendipity

Serendipity will help one to jump out of a rut, as well as improve the quality of one's meditation. This was one of the only times we looked at the essence's astrological birthchart, as Peter felt we should. There is a strong Uranian aspect to this essence, which is why it has this 'ready-to-jump' quality.

Paphiopedilum Predacious is a primary cross of *Paph. adductum* x *glanduliferum*

Settling with a Smile

Settling with a Smile helps the digestive system, by strengthening the etheric lining of the stomach and the gall bladder. It brings a quiet joy as well, hence the name.

Paph. Gold Dollar is a cross of *Paph. armeniacum* x *primulinum*

Sacral Release

Sacral Release Two of our customers have said that this gave them the most powerful essence experience they ever had. Pretty remarkable when you consider that I had bought it from a local garden centre! When Heather saw it in bloom her face glowed with the beauty of the orchid greeting her. Peter was with us, and said to Heather, "This one's for you!".

Note the way in which the blooms suggest the shape of vertebrae. In Adrian's TEK kit this is a major essence. It relates to blockages in the pelvic region, which occur more frequently in women than in men. The pelvis is the fundamental source of power within us, the universal energy which flows through the 1st & 2nd chakras. When the mind becomes entrenched in fear, guilt, anger and shame associated with sexuality, it can 'shut down' the pelvis, stopping the flow of pelvic energy - the pelvis becomes 'dead'. Sacral Release clears important levels of these blockages.

Try to buy orchids which give their full botanical name, and don't lose the tag like I did! After much sleuthing, I believe that this is the hybrid *Dendrobium Prapin* which was registered by the Chao Praya Orchid Nursery in Thailand in 1993.

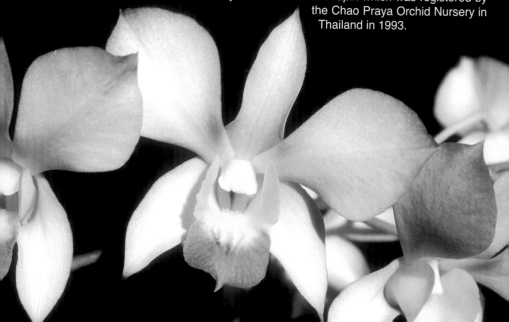

Serene Overview

In our society there is generally an under-valuing of women as they mature; in the West this has gone on for many centuries. This happens outwardly as well as inwardly, and it is the inner dynamic which Serene Overview helps to address.

Peter's name for this essence was "Devata", which is a Sanskrit word meaning the spiritual potential of the feminine aspect of the soul. And this essence conveys those qualities: serene, noble, ready to act with integrity but without force, and from the perspective of the wisdom that comes after many challenges over many years.

Heather saw herself as an eagle, soaring a mile high over the landscape below. Serene Overview helps us to see the landscape of our lives differently, and to act with serenity and grace from that higher perspective.

Comparetia speciosa is from the cloud-forests of Ecuador. Not a large plant, the blooms shown above are more or less life-size.

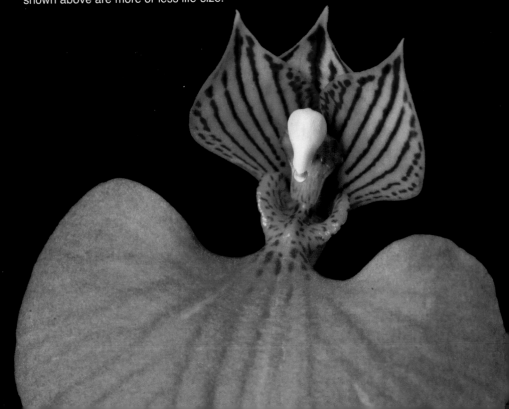

Secret Wisdom

Perhaps I should not admit to having favourites amongst the orchids, but this orchid and its essence hold a special place in my heart.

While there are several of the orchid essences which are especially suited to take whilst meditating, this is one which in my view should *only* be taken with the intention to meditate. This is not a remedy; this essence is all about deep inner stillness. Secret Wisdom invites you into a space beyond time, where Being is no longer involved in Becoming. I remember one of our early 2-day seminars on the LTOE, how one person struggled to understand what the orchid essences were about, until we meditated for 20 minutes on Secret Wisdom. In that extraordinary stillness, he finally understood the special gifts of the orchids.

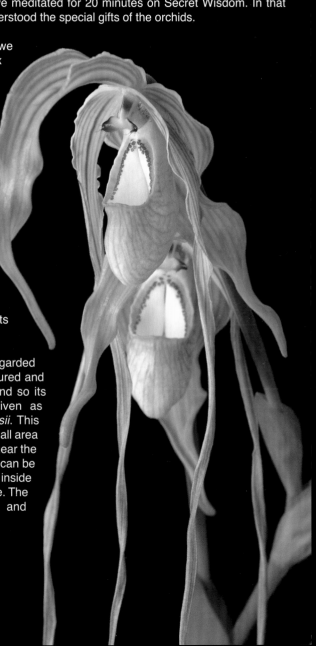

After we had made the essence, we held back from releasing it for six months, unsure if it was appropriate to bring an essence of such profound teaching into the hustle & bustle as it were of the 'marketplace'. And then one day, both Peter and I felt a shift, as if the orchid was letting us know that it was ok, that it was time...

Here more than anywhere else, words are utterly inadequate. There are some elements of our spiritual journey which cannot be verbalized, which can only be experienced. So disregard our descriptions when taking this essence, and allow yourself the time and space to hear the depth of its wisdom, the stillness of its being.

Phragmipedium wallisii is currently regarded as a variety of the much darker-coloured and larger *Phragmipedium caudatum*, and so its botanical name at this time is given as *Phragmipedium caudatum var. wallisii*. This is a terrestrial, and is found only in small area of southern Ecuador where it grows near the banks of the Rio Zamora. The petals can be nearly 20" (50 cm) in length, and the inside lobes of the pouch are porcelain-white. The blooms can last for over a month, and appear simultaneously.

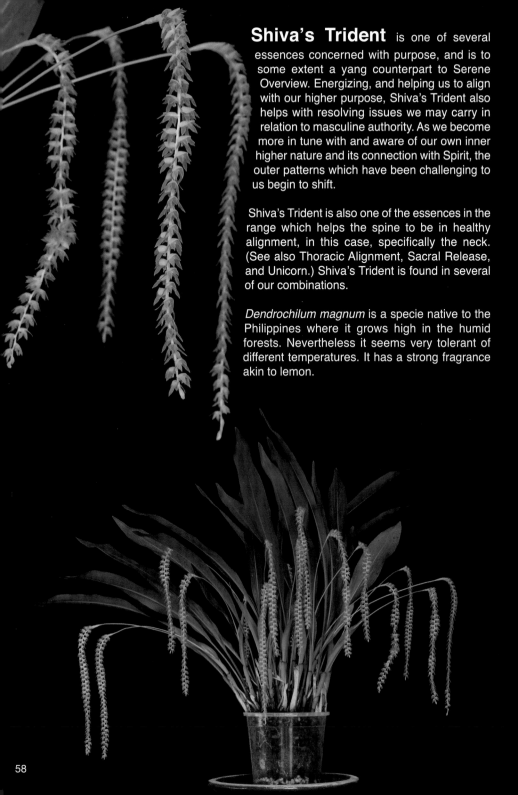

Shiva's Trident is one of several essences concerned with purpose, and is to some extent a yang counterpart to Serene Overview. Energizing, and helping us to align with our higher purpose, Shiva's Trident also helps with resolving issues we may carry in relation to masculine authority. As we become more in tune with and aware of our own inner higher nature and its connection with Spirit, the outer patterns which have been challenging to us begin to shift.

Shiva's Trident is also one of the essences in the range which helps the spine to be in healthy alignment, in this case, specifically the neck. (See also Thoracic Alignment, Sacral Release, and Unicorn.) Shiva's Trident is found in several of our combinations.

Dendrochilum magnum is a specie native to the Philippines where it grows high in the humid forests. Nevertheless it seems very tolerant of different temperatures. It has a strong fragrance akin to lemon.

Shadow Warrior has an unusual story behind its coming to be made. I initially only learnt of the existence of this orchid whilst browsing the web one night, and I had a clear high white dot about finding this orchid and making an essence with it. As my dots rarely commented on my seeking of orchids, this stood out as exceptional. So I contacted one of the semi-commercial orchids growers I know in England, who then a few months later let me know that he had located one in Germany I could have, if I still wanted it. After it settled into our greenhouse that spring, in then came into bloom that July. Adrian happened to arrive for a short break, and exclaimed when he saw this orchid in bloom that he had been searching for years for an essence that would address what this orchid's energy would address.

Adrian was very clear that the essence-making needed to take place largely in the dark, at night. The shutters of the room were closed, so in the morning only a small amount of light came into the room (through the heart-shaped holes in the shutters). As with Vital Core, the darkness of the space helped the essence to have greater access to our shadow aspect.

The human psyche carries an exceptionally powerful and subtle shadow which is capable of altering the journey of the soul into the light. The shadow is responsible for self-destructive, negative or ego-motivated beliefs and actions. When over-active the shadow interacts negatively with our core archetypes (personality traits) bringing out our worst qualities. An over-active shadow is a significant barrier to healing.

Shadow warrior acts to bring the shadow & light into equilibrium (we must acknowledge and accept the shadow within ourselves but it should not rule). It clears inner vision bringing about a change in perception whereby we connect with a deeper reality, aiding the soul's journey.

Bulbophyllum phalaenopsis is native to Borneo, and is one of a small section within the genus with very large leaves, and inflorescences which stink. To my nose the odour of Bulbophyllum phalaenopsis is akin the that from the bottom of a birdcage. The leaves are thick and fleshy, and can be nearly a meter long. The inflorescence is about the size of a large grapefruit.

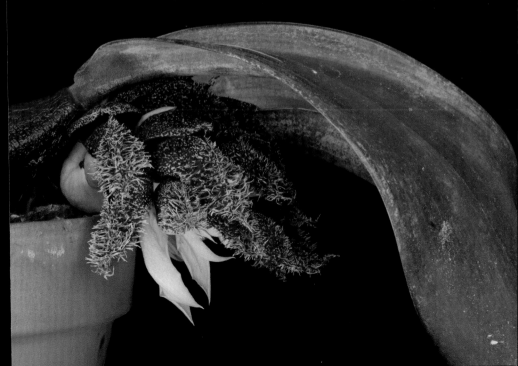

Source of Life

Our most recently made essence (February 2010), this had a very interesting genesis. Adrian had been hoping we would find the final energetic elements for his Therapeutic Energy Kinesiology kit when I made Base Regulator in early February, but wonderful as Base Regulator is, there was a need for a further orchid essence to be made to create the necessary energetic composition. Walking into the greenhouse, Adrian felt this delightful and delicate specie from Peru calling out to him. We brought the orchid out of the greenhouse, and set it up in a room in the house, with the bowl of water placed under the blooms.

It is best to take this essence in the morning, as it has a strong awakening quality. This is not to say it is at all like coffee! The effect is more subtle, and comes about slowly. A gentle yet insistent alertness persisted with both of us for many hours that night after we had sipped the mother tincture. The most noticeable, even palpable effect of sipping the mother tincture was what felt like a fine and cool spray starting from area of the perinium, felt very clearly for several inches down the insides of the thighs. Adrian was delighted, as he could sense that this essence completed the search he had been on for his TEK kit. When combined with Base Regulator and one other essence, it created a powerful composition we have called Sacral Regulator.

Adrian in his notes said: the essence is unique in being the only orchid essence which has an obvious selective target of the sexual aspect of the Dan Tien point and part of the 2nd chakra. It seems to enhance the sensitivity of the skin on the inside of the thighs' "sex skin". It realigns the energy systems in the pelvis, it rejuvenates the feeling of being alive in the pelvis, and 're-lights' the sexual centres to be aware of the deeper nature of ones sexuality. This essence needs to be bottled in the very dark purple Miron glass bottles.

Cochlioda beyrodtiana is an epiphyte found in the cool cloud-forests of Peru and Ecuador, which grows at roughly 2,200 meters. See also *Cochlioda noezliana* (Just Me). There are only eight species of Cochlioda.

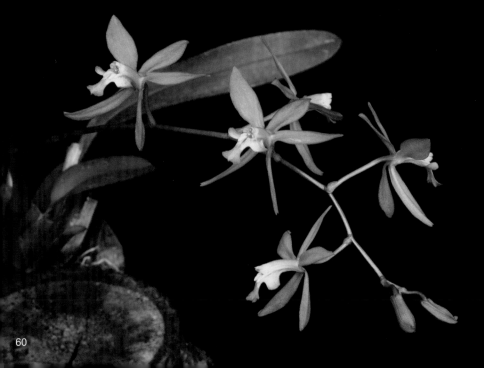

Spirit of the Higher Heart

is the same essence as Healing the Higher Heart, but without the addition of the 24 kt Gold essence. As with the other version of this orchid's essence, Spirit of the Higher Heart also helps to heal the Higher Heart chakra, but takes the action to a further level. So in general it will be best to use Healing the Higher Heart first for a week or two, and then follow it up with Spirit of the Higher Heart for even deeper healing.

This essence has a strong relationship with the spiritual chamber of the heart (see TOL5 notes) and the heart chakra. It is about unconditional love and unconditional acceptance of yourself and others. This is a much higher form of love than that of the heart chakra alone which relates to the ability to love. The essence acts to release the heart from emotional blocks, either karmic or current.

This is a vandaceous hybrid called *Vascostylis Roll on Red*, which was registered by the Brighton Orchid Nursery in Australia in 2004. *Vascostylis Roll on Red* is a cross of *Vascostylis Crownfox Red Gem* and *Ascocenda Peggy Foo*. Due to the large, long and vigorous roots it is common for these to be grown without bark, hanging in the air as seen here.

Songline
When we meditated on the mother tincture, Heather saw herself walking very very slowly along the bottom of a very narrow gorge, wide enough for only one person. Perplexed by the image, and by the treacle pace, she asked her guide what this signified. Unusually, he gave a full and direct reply: this image was about the soul's unique spiritual path, that path which is yours and yours alone. And it was to emphasize the importance of us putting even one foot forward on that path in our life, and the difficulty we find in doing so. We are so easily distracted from our deepest inner journey.

Paphiopedilum Honey is a primary hybrid (meaning both parents are species) made by crossing *Paph. primulinum* and *Paph. philippinense*.

Thoracic Alignment was made after several people in a seminar group noticed a strong shower of energy coming down from the plant, even though there was no bloom.

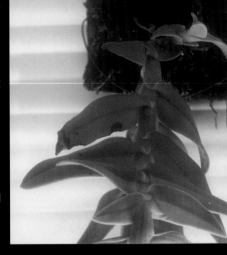

This essence is especially concerned with correct skeletal alignment of the thoracic region, to enable the healthy flow of energy within the body. This in turn enables our meditations to be deeper and more inspiring.

Very useful for massage and body-work in general.

Nanodes medusae is native to the cool cloud forests of the mountains of Ecuador.

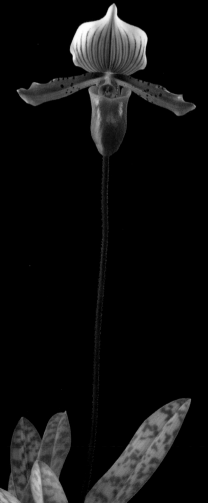

Totem helps you to connect with your animal spirit guides. There is a quality of quiet stillness and calm patience with this essence, and to experience its gift it is best to mirror those qualities within yourself by taking it in meditation. Close your eyes once you have had the drops, and see which animal comes to mind straight away.

This essence was one of two in the line made by Dominic Jones with Heather DeCam. Dominic had asked if he could help make an orchid essence, and so once Heather & I discussed it, the two of them went to the greenhouse. Out of perhaps 15 different orchids in bloom this was the one which called to Dominic. The upright stillness and strength of the orchid are qualities of soul found also in Dominic. And this is a part (for me) of the wonderful mystery of our small team at work in this project. For while I had bought the orchid at a show, and had been caring for it through the months, it took Dominic to feel that special resonance with it, so that an essence came to be made. I believe there is a certain strength in having some diversity in our approach to the orchids.

Paphiopedilum William Mathews 'Knobcreek' is an awarded hybrid. (The 'Knobcreek' portion of the name indicates that the plant has been awarded at an "official" show.)

Unicorn is an essence of tremendous physical focus. In meditation on the mother tincture Heather found herself engaged in a vigorous Kendo practice fight with her guide, with them sparring with wooden swords for over 10 minutes. For Peter this essence reminded him of a master Judo instructor he knew, who had that 'invincibility' of inner focus which is the key to victory in martial arts.

Though this essence can help with mental focus, its action is more fully on the physical level. If one is clumsy, Unicorn will help. For anyone engaged in any sports, from tennis to rugby or football, this essence can provide a welcome boost. Use it with New Vitality, Shiva's Trident and Vital Core to have a keenly focused energy boost. Unicorn also eases tension in the 7th cervical vertebrae, at the base of the neck. Such C7 tensions can give rise to tension headaches.

Gongora dresslerri is a specie native to Central America and Colombia, and has a pungent fragrance by day similar to the spice known as allspice.

Please see the close-up photo later in this book.

Unconditional Snuggles grabbed Natalie's attention in the greenhouse one day, at which point there was no question but the essence needed to be made. This essence is more than simply reassurring and comforting; in Dr. Brito-Babapulle's advanced kinesiology it is one of the 18 key essences for healing.

Combines very effectively with White Beauty to help with children's night-fears.

Paphiopedilum Snowbird is a "complex" hybrid. This term refers to hybridizing efforts that go back several decades, aiming to create larger, broader petaled Paphiopedilums. To my eye, these often look too forced, too unrelated to nature for my liking. Paph. Snowbird is lovely, but for the most part the complex Paphs do not appeal to me. And yet for many orchid growers, they are considered exceptionally desirable. I cannot help but wonder if the goals of orchid hybridizing would shift if orchid growers in general became aware of the energetic aspects of the plants.

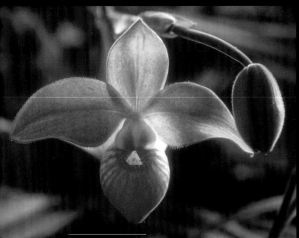

Unveiling Affection

is one of the loveliest and most extraordinary essences in the line, despite being the very first. Most people will experience the essence as a warm glow in their heart, and find that it helps them to not only open their heart with affection to the world around them, but also to love themselves. This secondary quality came about because of the slow opening of the bud (like the one shown here) during the hours of the essence-making.

Picture the bud opening, and the loving, affectionate energy of the bloom is being largely held within the bud, reflecting it back on itself. And so with the essence, we learn both to open our hearts to others, and also to have some of that affection reflected back within, to nurture ourselves. Self-love is not an easy lesson for most of us to learn, but this essence is an enormous help.

The gentle power of this essence is seen most fully with people who have been victims of sexual abuse in childhood. If such a person is within a supportive group environment (such as the seminars I teach), then usually their response is to burst into tears within 10 seconds of being given a few drops of Unveiling Affection. And in every single instance I have witnessed such a response, it has emerged that they did indeed have that trauma in childhood. The tears are brought on because the armour plating they have worn over their heart chakra for 30 or 50 years has suddenly melted, and their heart is deeply open for the first time since they were very young. This is a powerful experience, and should be supported with other essences and processes as well. Learning to live with our hearts open to the world after deep emotional and physical torment is a great challenge, but this orchid knows we are capable of deep healing and fundamental recovery.

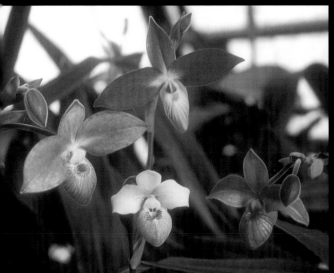

Phragmipedium Hanne Popow is a hybrid cross of two species: *Phrag. besseae* (top of photo, and also on the page opposite) and *Phrag. schlimii* (pink with white petals, bottom middle).

On the left-hand side of the photo is *Phrag. St. Ouen*, which is a cross of *Phrag. besseae* and *Phrag. Hanne Popow* (seen on the lower right of the photo). *Phragmipedium St. Ouen* produced the essence Golden Radiance.

Vital Core is of help at two related yet distinct levels. On a physical level it is an extraordinary energizer, helping to awaken all three of the lower chakras. It is very energizing of the gall bladder meridian, to the degree that people report waking up hungry in the morning after taking this essence, more so than in many years.

At another level it helps to bring light to the hidden shadows of our lower chakras, to help restore natural wholeness and health within them. This is a bit like spring-cleaning a pond, clearing the muck which has gathered... Vital Core was made largely in the dark, at the orchid's request, with the beams of a rising full moon shining on the orchid and the bowl of water through a break in the curtains. Only once it had been made did we understand its request: that by being made largely in the dark, it would have better access to our own shadow side.

This essence was made the same weekend in November as Celestial Siren, and these two form a type of yin-yang pair. Vital Core works at levels beyond that of Sacral Release; it can be a good idea to work with the latter first, and then to follow up with some days of Vital Core.

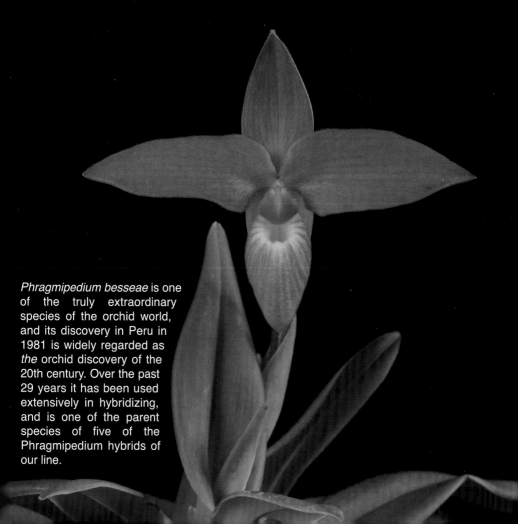

Phragmipedium besseae is one of the truly extraordinary species of the orchid world, and its discovery in Peru in 1981 is widely regarded as *the* orchid discovery of the 20th century. Over the past 29 years it has been used extensively in hybridizing, and is one of the parent species of five of the Phragmipedium hybrids of our line.

Walking to the Earth's Rhythm was made a few weeks after Heather and I had made Guardian of the Inner Journey, and it was very clear that these two were a kind of pair. When meditating on Guardian of the Inner Journey it is quite possible to be left rather ungrounded, and so it is best to then take Walking to the Earth's Rhythm for its gentle grounding energy.

Walking to the Earth's Rhythm is quietly joyful, very gently grounding, and deeply dignified. One example of its use would be when a client has done some powerful or deep emotional releasing, then this essence would be one to seriously consider giving them before they leave your treatment room.

With all of our involvement with technology these days, we are in grave danger of losing our sense of connection with the Earth and her rhythms. This essence helps to address this challenge, to help us move forward in harmony with the Earth.

The following is Adrian's description of the action of this essence, based on his kinesiological work with it.

This essence helps release us from being 'trapped' in negative beliefs and the negative archetypes (or personalities) within us. It has a strong relationship with Shadow warrior and when that fails to clear the shadow this essence may be needed.

The trapped receptor related to this essence is a minor chakra on the left shoulder associated with the physical manifestation of the shadow. It is a point of emotional lock related to the negative aspects of the four survival archetypes. These archetypes are:

The Prostitute - usually in a financial sense, a reflection of the Mercedes Benz culture in which we put money or power above our spiritual journey.

The Victim, in who instead of using difficult experiences to move forward in the souls journey, suffering has become its identity.

The Child, an easily recognised archetype where childhood experiences clouds interaction with the world.

The Saboteur, probably one of the most potent archetypes in which fear of failure (or success) holds the person back from achieving their potential.

It is important to be familiar with the representation of these four archetypes. The shadow aspect is very seductive and allows escape from emotional or spiritual reality either into self-destructive behaviour or over-identification with the 'ego'.

The visualization correction that aids this essence represents the fact that the patient is not 'trapped' in a rigid structure such as a box but instead in a tunnel in the darkness (which represents fear) with a 'way out' into the rose pink light which represents love. Imagine yourself in a dark tunnel walking slowly towards a rose pink light in the distance, which comes to surround you. Breathe this rose pink light in and out three times.

Paphipedilum St. Swithin is a remarkable primary hybrid, a cross of *Paph. rothschildianum* and *Paph. philippinense*. With a striking air of dignity and beauty, it draws gasps of admiration when in bloom in the greenhouse. I took this photo the day after the essence was made, using a 600mm lens; it remains one of my favourites of all my orchid photographs.

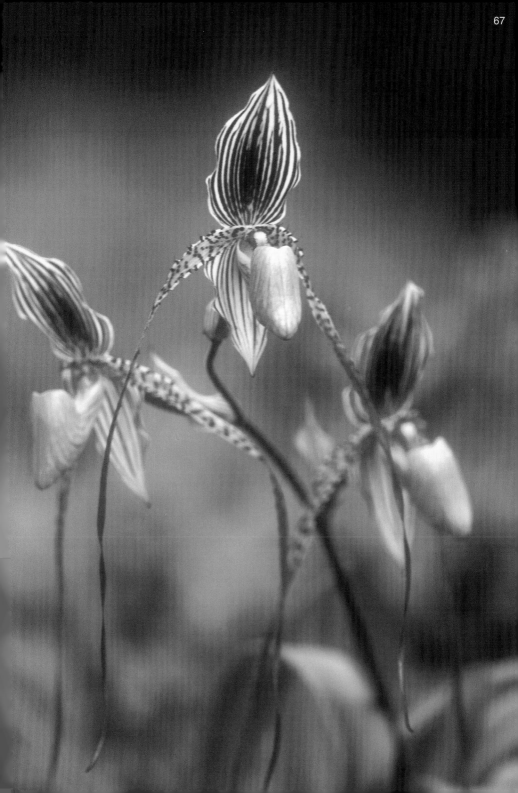

White Beauty

White Beauty was made with a heart-shaped piece of rose quartz sitting in the bowl of water, so this essence conveys both the beautiful, loving energy of the orchid, as well as the heart-nurturing qualities of rose quartz. Made in early 1999, we very soon tried putting this essence into a spray bottle, with rose otto oil added for fragrance. We found it to be wonderfully de-stressing and calming, with a gently nurturing and loving energy entering the crown chakra.

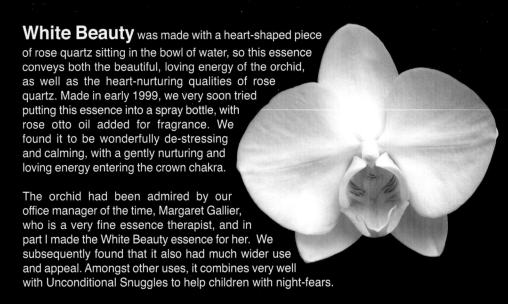

The orchid had been admired by our office manager of the time, Margaret Gallier, who is a very fine essence therapist, and in part I made the White Beauty essence for her. We subsequently found that it also had much wider use and appeal. Amongst other uses, it combines very well with Unconditional Snuggles to help children with night-fears.

Phalaenopsis aphrodite is a specie from the Philippines region up to Taiwan, and is very similar to *Phal. amabilis* - usually only experts are able to distinguish the two species.

Wingéd Gold

Wingéd Gold is a wonderful essence for creative writing, the multitude of golden blooms appearing to signify the fecundity of the imagination. It is also one of the essences in our range to help us be in tune with our deeper purpose in the flow of our lives (see also Andean Fire, Life Direction and Songline). Both of these aspects of the essence can be understood further in noting the chakras it primarily resonates with: the Inner Chamber of the Heart, the Ajana centre, and the Crown chakra.

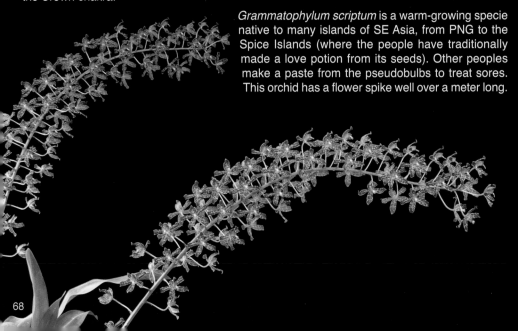

Grammatophylum scriptum is a warm-growing specie native to many islands of SE Asia, from PNG to the Spice Islands (where the people have traditionally made a love potion from its seeds). Other peoples make a paste from the pseudobulbs to treat sores. This orchid has a flower spike well over a meter long.

Wisdom of Compassion called out to Heather in the greenhouse, "Make an essence with me, I'm about Compassion". And so we made the essence, learning only later that it was made on the Tibetan anniversary of the Buddha's enlightenment. This essence conveys a deep teaching to one's heart, about the nature of loving compassion. The heart becomes a broad river flowing gently out to the world, embracing the pain and suffering yet without one's heart suffering in the process. The heart acknowledges the suffering, and yet understands a deeper reality of Being underlying it. The heart's river of Compassion becomes in itself a blessing on all beings. We would wish for this essence to be shared with as many people as possible, to transform humanity's relationship with itself.

Phalaenopsis Sussex Silk is a stunningly beautiful fourteenth generation hybrid.

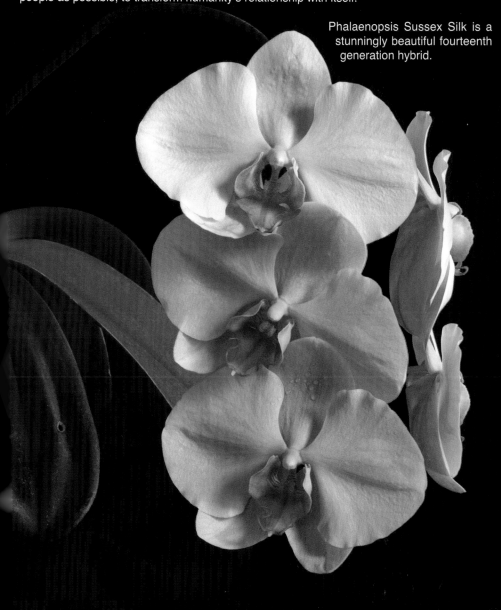

Combination Essences

To date we have created 18 combinations with the LTOE, more than a decade since we started making the essences themselves. From one perspective, this does not seem like a large number, since well over a billion combinations are possible with the 62 single essences we have at this point. However, as a general rule we caution against 'simply' combining the orchid essences, as they have such depth to their nature that the results are not straight-forward. Use discernment and intuition, and verify that the result is what you may be looking for. Combining is not a neutral action energetically, and best results requires care and attention. The ones we have created are described in the following pages. They are listed only partially alphabetically, as certain ones make more sense to describe on the same page.

Active Serenity

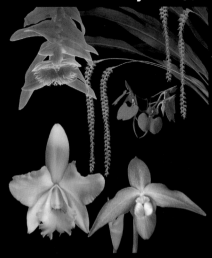

Acting primarily on the mental body centres, this combination is excellent for di-stress and fatigue. Tension held in the brain stem and alta major chakra (back of the head) is dissolved. Provides relief in the frontal lobes, aiding critical thinking & decision making. The crown chakra opens to a new clarity and mental energy which is calm yet energized. An excellent essence to use in times of major life transitions.

This is almost the same combination as Happy Relief, but the addition of Serene Overview brings a strongly serene quality to the essence. When feeling low, take Active Serenity straight from the bottle, and then two minutes later take drops of Happy Relief. It is very important that the two essences are taken in this order, because the serene quality of Active Serenity would dramatically counter the 'happy' effect of the other combination. Far better to end on a happy note!

Happy Relief

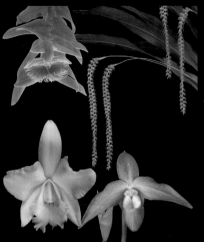

Brings a sense of happiness & gentle yet strong vitality. Helps one to feel quietly happy, and at the same time clearing mental or emotional tension, and clears stress from the limbic centre in the brain. The Ba-hui point opens to give the head a sense of upward lift. A very good relief remedy in challenging situations.

When we first made this combination, we were surprised to find that it brought a smile to the lips of almost everyone who tried it. Our surprise was because this quality is not found in any of the four orchids which make it. This is a very clear (and positive) example of our point that combining the orchid essences is not a neutral action, that the sum is at the very least different from all of the parts.

As indicated above, highly recommended for anyone who is feeling down, but they should take Active Serenity drops first.

Being Present

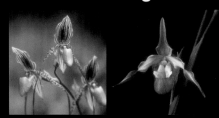

Helps one to be present wherever one is. Very good to use after a long journey, to assist all the parts of one's body and mind to 'arrive'. Good for jet lag, as the Being in Time component brings one's body cycles into harmony with the cycles of nature of the new time zone. Also helpful for both parties in facing difficult issues in conversation.

Gentle Geisha

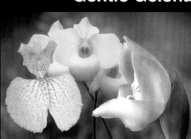

Energetically almost the opposite of Double Espresso, this combination is excellent for unwinding at the end of the day. Helps to calm the overly-active mind, bringing one very gently, graciously back into one's body. Imagine sinking one's head down into a soft silk cushion, setting aside concern for one's many responsibilities and cares for a while. Allow the energies of these three beautiful orchids to soothe and nurture you, while you relax with a cup of tea...

Gentle Sleep

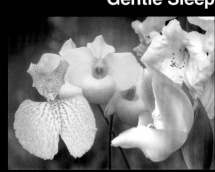

Gentle Sleep is an enhanced version of Gentle Geisha, with the addition of the essence of Rhododendron griffithianum, made by Don in Achamore Gardens. Rhod. griffithianum is a deeply calming, relaxing and peaceful essence. This 4th component is not an orchid essence, but these days, especially in the UK, disturbed sleep has become a major issue for many, and so the importance of 'bending' our tradition in this one instance felt appropriate. Gentle Sleep helps one to achieve a deeper and more relaxed sleep.

Healing the Hidden

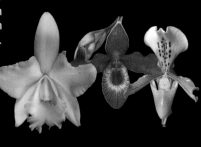

The three essences in this combination work together as a team, rather than as a blend. We had never encountered this before: each essence arrives in turn when you take the drops, and will be experienced in the appropriate order for your needs at that moment. It was Natalie who worked out that the inclusion of Andean Fire was what brought about this unusual quality, owing to its deep sense of purpose.

If you are in tears, Heyoka will bring relief; if you are hiding tears, Heyoka will remind you that you are carrying that pain and grief. What we hide from others for long eventually becomes hidden to ourselves.

Double Espresso

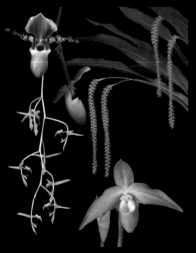

A very yang combination for those times when one needs an extra yang boost to one's energy. An essence equivalent to a cup of strong java, not to be taken daily or frequently, but rather in critical instances when extra energy is urgently required.

This essence is not unlike an essence equivalent to ginseng, and we would emphasize that it is best used sparingly. However, one good use of it would be in competitive sports, where it will give the athlete an extra boost. Depending on the body type, Vital Lift would be a good alternate, which would also be the better essence for training.

Vital Lift

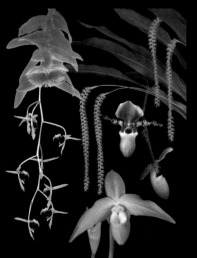

This combination is the same as Double Espresso, but with the aligning & calming energy brought by Core of Being. Gives one a calm and centred boost of energy. Helpful when one is flagging, giving stamina for focused work. Useful as an adjunct to training for athletes.

The impact of Core of Being in this combination is very interesting. Whereas Double Espresso is likely to make one want to jump out of your chair and get going, Vital Lift has a quality of being more centered and contained - all due to the addition of Core of Being.

A useful approach for athletes would be to use Vital Lift when training, and then Double Espresso when the match is on, and the game is running.

Party Time!

A celebration of the sensual dance of life. To everything there is a time and purpose, and with this essence we can remember fun, and the enjoyment of the senses. Dance again, lest you forget the joy it brings!

One customer found that this essence lifted her spirits, so even on a rainy winter day, she was focused on the beauty of church bells ringing, rather than on the negative thoughts and feelings which had been troubling her before.

Clearing & Releasing

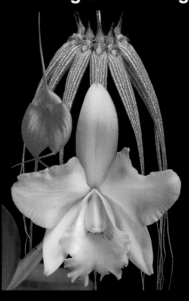

We had initially thought of the Angelic Canopy spray as all the space clearing help one might need, until we encountered one person on a seminar who needed deeper help. Clearly if there is a karmic aspect to the energies, then that needs to be addressed: and so Releasing Karmic Patterns was added. Pushing Back the Night has very high reach, and brings a high alignment of energy. With all 3 essences combined, this is a very powerful energy cleanser, a bit like an interior spring cleaning for the psyche and soul.

If a person has played around with so-called "recreational drugs", or had a drug habit, then this combination will help to rid their aura of any low-level astral forms which may have entered their weakened aura. Soul Shield will then help to strengthen the aura and help to repair it.

Also very popular now in the aura spray form.

Soul Shield

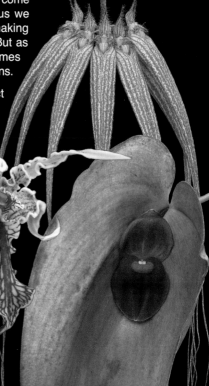

It came as a shock to Heather & I one day when during a meditation on one of the orchid essences, a being as black as the night sky entered the room, and told Heather he had "come from the Sun" and that he had come in order to tell us we needed to protect ourselves. Surely we were just making delightful orchid essences, a quite innocent activity? But as time went by, we came to understand that there are times when we need to protect ourselves, for a variety of reasons.

People that work with light are highly likely to attract strong challenges from diverse and sometimes dark energies from time to time. There is also the global situation, which is increasingly shrouded in dark and threatening shadows. Soul Shield provides powerful protection at multiple levels, to help us bring that light we carry within safely through with strength and certainty.

Also helps to strengthen the auric field when taken daily for several weeks, so that one is not so susceptible to the incursions of electromagnetic radiations (such as the UK's ubiquitous Tetra masts) which may be interfering with one's sleep parttern. In such situations, best used in conjunction with Gentle Sleep or Sleep of Peace, as well as Being in Time.

Sacral Regulator

Sacral Regulator is a combination of three essences: Core Release, Source of Life and an essence called Child's Play. This latter essence was made by Rose Titchiner in Norfolk, England as part of her Light Heart Essences range. She stopped producing and selling her essences in 2009 for health reasons, but the Child's Play essence had been so vital to Adrian's work for several years that he bought the mother tiuncture, and arranged for it to be sent to us at IFER, for us to bottle, so there could be a continued supply. Along with Vital Core, Unveiling Affection, Unconditional Snuggles and Sacral Release, Child's Play has been a key energetic tool for Adrian in correcting blockages and imbalances in the pelvic pulsation points and receptors. Not a flower essence, Child's Play is one of what Rose referred to as her "Intentional" essences. There is a lightness and innocence to this essence which Adrian has found to be exceptionally potent in his Therapeutic Energy Kinesiology.

This combination does what the sum of the parts would be in that it acts on the 1st, 2nd, 3rd, 6th and 7th chakras; it is purifying of the liver and also produces an increased sense of wellbeing and comfort within the pelvic region after a period of disturbance. On testing the essence it is clear that it has a marked effect on both levels of the dead pelvis syndrome, and does start the process of renewing and regeneration of the Gate of Life.

We should explain that the term "dead pelvis syndrome" is used by Adrian for a set of energetic conditions he frequently finds in his work, whereby various of the receptors and pulsation points in the pelvic area are blocked or suppressed. Please see his chart in the second half of this book for an illustration of the points, and the essences he uses to re-balance these points.

Outside of the kinesiological descriptions, one is likely to find that Sacral Regulator gives a sense of wellbeing, emanating from the pelvic area, and at the same time an expanded awareness around the head. Sexuality moves away from 'performance' to intimacy and deep communion.

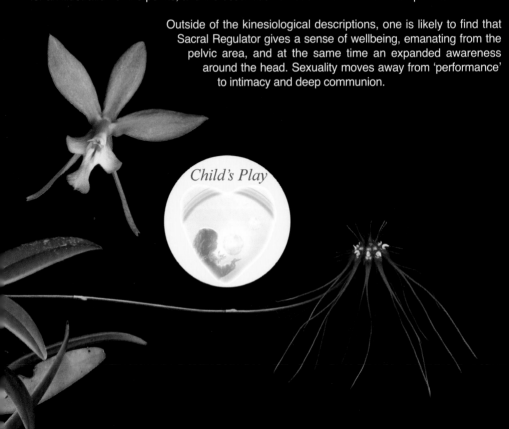

Child's Play

Sleep of Peace

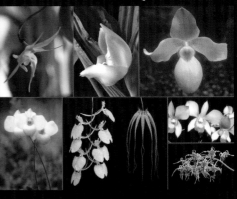

Sleep of Peace helps to promote deeper and longer-lasting sleep, but in a different manner from Gentle Sleep. This combination was created by Dr. Jessica Middleton, who found it helped her sleep pattern considerably. More research on this combination was then done by Dr. Brito-Babapulle and IFER, to find its optimum potency, as well as to try to understand more fully how it helps our sleep.

Sleep of Peace appears to help with our processing of memories, so that the mind is able to process data from the day more efficiently while one is asleep. After a few days of use it appears to bring about deep processing & shifting of old memories which are 'gathering dust' and interfering with the efficient processing of the daily data. It is this jumble of old memories, traumas and fears which are often a significant part of the picture of disturbed sleep patterns. In general it is best to take Sleep of Peace for no more than one week at a time, as the new pattern of deeper sleep is able to carry on without the essence. Taking a drop at bedtime once every week or two thereafter should suffice.

Whether Sleep of Peace or Gentle Sleep will be the best help for a given individual will depend on their circumstances, character etc. Also see Soul Shield in relation to sleep patterns and one's exposure to electro-magnetic fields.

Shiva's Crown

Heightens and deepens the soul's understanding of its journey in this physical body. This essence goes into a part of the brain known as the limbic system and connects the causal body with the soul's journey and its divine contract, thus enhancing the process of spiritual healing. Assists in the therapeutic effects of other healing processes in the body as well. May be used in conjunction with Sleep of Peace to help with one's sleep patterns.

On a somewhat technical note, Shiva's Crown connects the dreaming point on the top of the head with two points on the temporal axis the right and left, the left being the shadow side of the energy system.

A powerful essence for deep meditations.

Temple of Light

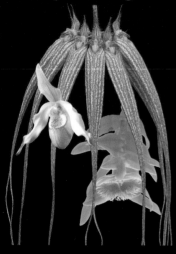

Temple of Light (5)

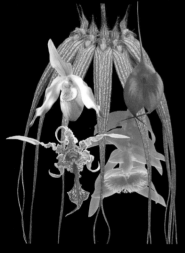

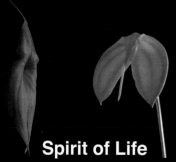

Spirit of Life

Temple of Light was created to address an incongruity which may arise between the Ba-hui point and the Inner Chamber of the Heart chakra, and the 7th & 4th chakras as well. Adrian's experience is that there is no real healing when these four points are not properly connected. To assist a rapid resolution of this problem, this essence was called into being. The activity of the essence is as follows: The first effect starts at the brow or Ajna chakra, then draws around the head & upwards to pull on and thus open the Ba-hui point and continues on a vertical route. This is the joint effort of Core of Being, which is a powerful activator, and Pushing Back the Night, which tells the causal body that there is no darkness left to fear.

Renewing Life's influence on both the root and 12th chakras creates a grounding of the spirit, which again invites the Inner Chamber of the Heart to open. The Inner Chamber is often the way to reconnect to the Divine. But in the case of those traditions which have abandoned the inner sacred feminine, a "reverse order" approach arises, i.e. going to the outer limits of Spiritual Reality and from that depth & intensity the effort is made to provide the protection & space for the delicate inner temple to be built. As a prolonged effort this approach tends to create the disconnection described above. Renewing Life indirectly calls on the inner chamber to position itself as the inner temple now that any negative energies have been evicted from the immediate vicinity. So this remedy invites the feminine to accept and then later challenge those big belief systems wherein God lives exclusively outside of the temple of the body and is always just out of reach of the inner chamber, or the Chalice of the Spirit.

Some people are unable to readily allow the re-connections described above. What Adrian found is that there is a latent disconnection between the 6th, 7th and 8th chakras in these clients. We found that the addition of two essences to the Temple of Light combination solved the problem. By including Protective Presence, the matrix of the causal body more readily nurtures the body's chakras creating an inner strength to accept one's deepest inner being. As a karmic element is likely to be present as well, Releasing Karmic Patterns was added, which also shifts the 8th chakra into a harmonious relationship with the 7th chakra, allowing divine consciousness to inspire the crown chakra.

Please see the descriptions for Fire of Life and Furnace of Life earlier in this book for the description of the qualities of Spirit of Life.

Positive Flow

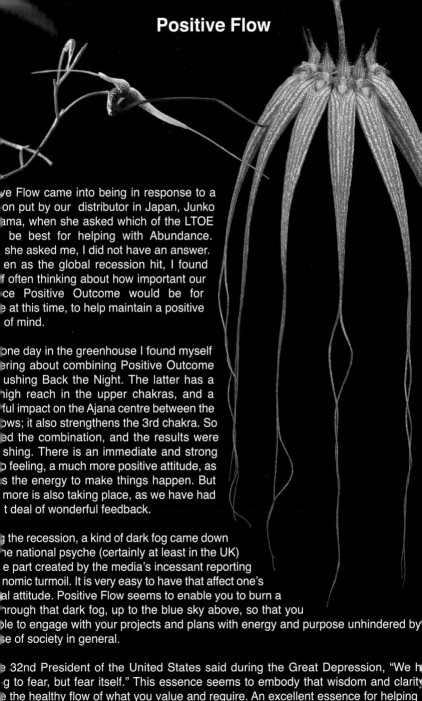

...ve Flow came into being in response to a ...on put by our distributor in Japan, Junko ...ama, when she asked which of the LTOE ... be best for helping with Abundance. ... she asked me, I did not have an answer. ...en as the global recession hit, I found ...f often thinking about how important our ...ce Positive Outcome would be for ...e at this time, to help maintain a positive ... of mind.

...one day in the greenhouse I found myself ...ering about combining Positive Outcome ... ushing Back the Night. The latter has a ...high reach in the upper chakras, and a ...ful impact on the Ajana centre between the ...ows; it also strengthens the 3rd chakra. So ...ed the combination, and the results were ...shing. There is an immediate and strong ...o feeling, a much more positive attitude, as ...s the energy to make things happen. But ...more is also taking place, as we have had ...t deal of wonderful feedback.

...g the recession, a kind of dark fog came down ...he national psyche (certainly at least in the UK) ...e part created by the media's incessant reporting ...nomic turmoil. It is very easy to have that affect one's ...al attitude. Positive Flow seems to enable you to burn a ...hrough that dark fog, up to the blue sky above, so that you ...le to engage with your projects and plans with energy and purpose unhindered by ...se of society in general.

...e 32nd President of the United States said during the Great Depression, "We h... ...g to fear, but fear itself." This essence seems to embody that wisdom and clarit... ...e the healthy flow of what you value and require. An excellent essence for helping ... projects under way, and to bring them to fruition.

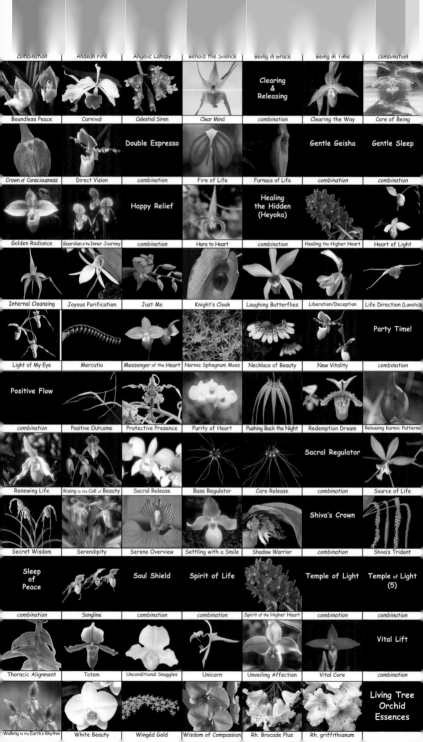

Andean Fire	Life Direction (Lanata)	Unicorn
Angelic Canopy	Light of my Eye	Unveiling Affection
Base Regulator	Mercutio	Vital Core
Behold the Silence	Messenger of the Heart	Walking to the Earth's Rhythm
Being in Time	Narnia Sphagnum Moss	White Beauty
Being in Grace	Necklace of Beauty	Wingéd Gold
Boundless Peace	New Vitality	Wisdom of Compassion
Carnival	Positive Outcome	Rhododendron Brocade Plus
Celestial Siren	Protective Presence	Rhododendron griffithianum
Clear mind	Purity of Heart	**Combination Essences (18)**
Clearing the Way	Pushing Back the Night	Active Serenity
Core of Being	Redemption Dream	Being Present
Core Release	Releasing Karmic Patterns	Clearing & Releasing
Crown of Consciousness	Renewing Life	Double Espresso
Direct Vision	Rising to the Call of Beauty	Gentle Geisha
Fire of Life	Sacral Release	Gentle Sleep
Furnace of Life	Secret Wisdom	Happy Relief
Guardian of the Inner Journey	Serendipity	Healing the Hidden (Heyoka)
Golden Radiance	Serene Overview	Party Time!
Hara to Heart	Settling with a Smile	Positive Flow
Healing the Higher Heart	Shadow Warrior	Sacral Regulator
Heart of Light	Shiva's Trident	Shiva's Crown
Internal Cleansing	Songline	Sleep of Peace
Joyous Purification	Source of Life	Soul Shield
Just me	Spirit of the Higher Heart	Spirit of Life
Knight's Cloak	Thoracic Alignment	Temple of Light
Laughing Butterflies	Totem	Temple of Light (5)
Liberation/Deception	Unconditional Snuggles	Vital Lift

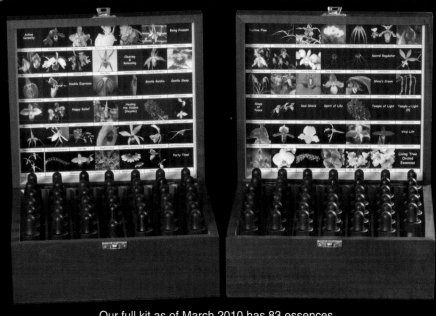

Our full kit as of March 2010 has 83 essences,
62 of which are single orchid essences, and 18 are combinations.
se note that all of our combinations as well as single essences are made at stock streng

Essence	Lung	Large Intestine	Stomach	Spleen	Heart	Small Intestine	Bladder	Kidney	Heart Protect.	Triple Warmer	Gall Bladder	Liver	Concept. Vessel	Govern. Vessel	Ming Men
Active Serenity					●				●						
Andean Fire								●					●		
Angelic Canopy								●							
Base Regulator				●								●			
Behold the Silence								●							
Being in Grace	●														
Being in Time								●			●				
Being Present			●						●						
Boundless Peace					●										
Carnival									●	●					
Celestial Siren								●					●		
Clear Mind	●													●	
Clearing & Releasing		●											●		
Clearing the Way /Self Belief						●								●	
Core of Being			●												
Core Release															
Crown of Consciousness										●			●		
Direct Vision	●								●						
Double Espresso					●										
Fire of Life	●														
Furnace of Life					●										●
Gentle Geisha						●					●				
Gentle Sleep	●							●							
Golden Radiance				●				●							
Guardian of the Inner Journey				●									●		
Happy Relief	●														
Hara to Heart					●										●
Healing the Hidden (Heyoka)	●														
Healing the Higher Heart					●								●		
Heart of Light					●					●					
Internal Cleansing								●			●	●			
Joyous Purification					●										
Just Me														●	
Knight's Cloak													●		●
Laughing Butterflies			●						●						
Liberation / Deception		●													
Life Direction (Lanata)	●									●					
Light of My Eye					●										
Mercutio							●								
Messenger of the Heart					●				●						

Lung	Lge. Intest.	Stomach	Spleen	Heart	Sml. Intest.	Bladder	Kidney	Hrt. Protect.	Trip. Warm.	Gall Bladder	Liver	Conc. Ves.	Gov. Ves.	Ming Men	Essence
						■									Narnia Sphagnum Moss
■								■							Necklace of Beauty
						■								■	New Vitality
		■											■		Party Time
									■				■		Positive Flow
	■										■				Positive Outcome
					■										Protective Presence
■				■											Purity of Heart
										■			■		Pushing Back the Night
	■														Redemption Dream
								■				■			Releasing Karmic Patterns
									■						Renewing Life
■															Rising to the Call of Beauty
	■														Sacral Regulator
							■						■		Sacral Release
			■												Secret Wisdom
	■						■								Serene Overview (Devata)
	■														Serendipity
				■											Settling with a Smile
			■											■	Shadow Facing
■															Shadow Warrior
			■												Shiva's Crown
				■			■								Shiva's Trident
								■	■						Sleep of Peace
								■							Songline
														■	Soul Shield
	■														Source of Life
							■								Spirit of Life
						■								■	Spirit of the Higher Heart
							■								Temple of Light
	■		■												Temple of Light (5)
		■			■										Thoracic Alignment
■					■										Totem
			■									■			Unconditional Snuggles
	■													■	Unicorn
			■			■									Unveiling Affection
						■				■					Vital Core
		■								■				■	Vital Lift
■															Walking to the Earth's Rhythm
								■					■		White Beauty
	■	■													Winged Gold
														■	Wisdom of Compassion

Essences chart — body point / chakra associations (columns are body points; each essence's Maker and markings shown).

Legend of body-point abbreviations: CB = Causal Body, DT = Dreamtime point, 7 = Crown Chakra, BP = Ba'hui point, 6 = Brow / 3rd Eye, AC = Ajana Centre, BTC = Back of Throat Chakra, 5 = Throat Chakra, ICH = Inner Chamber of the Heart chakra, ♥/4 = Heart Chakra, 3CB = 3rd Chakra Belt, 3 = Solar Plexus, 2 = Sacral Chakra, 1 = Root Chakra.

Essence	Maker	Root (1)	Sacral (2)	Solar Plexus (3)	3rd Chakra Belt	Heart	Inner Ch. Heart (ICH)	Throat (5)	Back of Throat (BTC)	Ajana (AC)	Brow (6)	Ba'hui (BP)	Crown (7)	Dreamtime (DT)	Causal Body (CB)	No.
Active Serenity	DD+HD			3			ICH	5			6		7	DT		
Andean Fire	DD+HD					♥										
Angelic Canopy	DD(+ABB)		2										7			
Base Regulator	DD+HD	1										BP				
Behold the Silence	DD+HD									AC	6		7	DT	CB	15
Being in Grace	DD+HD	1		3		♥							7			
Being in Time	DD+HD					♥										
Being Present	DD+HD	1	2			♥	ICH						7		CB	14
Boundless Peace	DD+HD		2	3	3CB	♥				AC					CB	
Carnival	DD+HD		2	3		♥				AC						10 11
Celestial Siren	DD+ABB		2			♥		5		AC			7			
Clear Mind	DD															
Clearing & Releasing	DD+HD	1														
Clearing the Way	DD+HD							5	BTC				7			
Core of Being	DD+HD	1		3		♥	ICH			AC	6		7	DT		13 14
Core Release	DD(+ABB)														CB	
Crown Consciousness	DD+HD				3CB	♥	ICH			AC			7	DT		
Direct Vision	DD+HD					♥	ICH			AC	6		7		CB	
Double Espresso	DD(+ABB)	1				♥							7			
Fire of Life	DD(+ABB)	1				♥	ICH			AC			7	DT	CB	
Furnace of Life	DD+HD					♥										
Gentle Geisha						♥					6					
Gentle Sleep						♥	ICH						7			
Golden Radiance	DD+HD					♥	ICH			AC			7	DT	CB	
Guardian of Inner J.	DD+HD	1				♥					6		7		CB	
Happy Relief	DD+HD		2		3CB	♥				AC		BP	7		CB	
Hara to Heart	DD+HD				3CB	♥							7			
Healing the Hidden	DD+HD				3CB	♥					6					
Healing High. Heart	DD+ABB					♥	ICH			AC			7			
Heart of Light	DD+ABB					♥	ICH						7			
Internal Cleansing	DD+HD					♥	ICH									
Joyous Purification	DD+HD							5	BTC							
Just Me	DD+NS					♥		5			6					
Knight's Cloak	HD+DJ					4		5					7			17
Laughing Butterflies	DD+HD			3		♥				AC	6					14
Liberation / Decep.	DD+NS	1	2	3						AC			7			
Life Direction	DD+NS		2			♥					6			DT		
Light of My Eye	DD+HD		2				ICH			AC	6		7			8 9 10

Bottom of table: "added 24 karat Gold essence" (combo / single).

2 means based on Peter Tadd's reading, where different from Linda Jeffrey's testing

	Name	1	2	3	3BC	4	ICH	5	BTC	AC	6	BP	7	AM	8	9	10	11	12	13	14	15	16	17	18	19	20	21	22	23	24	25	26	CB
DD	Messenger of Heart						ICH	5				BP																						
	Narnia Sphag. Moss																																	
DD+NS	Necklace of Beauty						ICH	5			6	BP																						
DD(+ABB)	New Vitality	1	2				ICH	5																										
	Party Time			3			ICH	5					7																						
	Positive Flow									AC				DT																				
DD+HD	Positive Outcome									AC			7	DT																				
DD+HD	Protective Presence			3						AC																								
DD+HD	Purity of Heart			3			ICH	5		AC			7																					
DD+HD	Pushing Back Night	1					ICH						7																					
DD	Redemption Dream						ICH				6		7																					
DD+HD	Releas. Karmic Patt.												7																					
DD+HD	Renewing Life						ICH	5		AC	6	BP	7																					
DD+HD	Rising Call of Beauty			3						AC				DT					12		14													
	Sacral Regulator		2				ICH		BTC																									
DD+HD	Sacral Release		2								6		7																					
DD+HD	Secret Wisdom						ICH				6						10																	
DD+HD	Serene Overview						ICH	5		AC	6		7	DT	8					13														
DD+HD	Serendipity		2					5			6			DT																				
DD+HD	Settling with a Smile	1								AC																								
DD+NS	Shadow Facing	1								AC			7																					
DD+ABB	Shadow Warrior	1		3							6	BP	7																					CB
	Shiva's Crown								BTC				7																					
DD+HD	Shiva's Trident										6	BP	7								13														
	Sleep of Peace							5			6		7																					CB
DD+HD	Songline	1					ICH			AC			7																					
DD+ABB	Soul Shield						ICH			AC																								
DD+ABB	Source of Life		2				ICH																											
	Spirit of Life	1	2																															
DD+ABB	Spirit of High. Heart						ICH			AC		BP		DT																				
	Temple of Light						ICH			AC																								
	Temple of Light (5)						ICH			AC																								
DD+HD	Thoracic Alignment	1						5		AC	6			DT																				
	Totem						ICH			AC			7							12														
HD+DJ	Uncond. Snuggles	1				4																												
DD+NS	Unicorn						ICH			AC	6		7																					
DD+HD	Unveiling Affection					4	ICH			AC				DT																				
DD (+PT)	Vital Core	1	2							AC		BP		DT																				
DD+ABB	Vital Lift		2	3									7																					
DD+HD	Walk. Earth's Rhythm	1					ICH			AC	6	BP		DT						13														
DD	White Beauty						ICH			AC		BP		DT																				
DD+HD	Winged Gold						ICH				6		7																					
DD+HD	Wisdom Compassion						ICH						7																					
		1	2	3	3BC	4	ICH	5	BTC	AC	6	BP	7	AM	8	9	10	11	12	13	14	15	16	17	18	19	20	21	22	23	24	25	26	CB

Aura Sprays are one of the forms in which people can experience the benefits of the essences, and whereas the drops work from the inside out, the sprays work directly on the auric field, shifting energies from the outside, moving in. Even people with no experience of essences can readily feel the effect of the sprays. Over the years though I had seen that people could be put off a good spray simply because of the fragrance the makers had chosen to enhance their spray didn't suit them. We therefore provide a choice of two different blends of essential oils for customers to choose between. Both are carefully chosen to be effective, while the differences of oils will provide very subtle differences in action on the aura.

Angelic Canopy Aura Spray

A delightful and calming spray for clearing the aura as well as office & living spaces of negative energies. Balm for the troubled soul, it nurtures those who are in grief, despair or who have lost hope. Good for rescue dogs. Very effective in space clearing as well as for aura cleansing.

This is probably our most universal aura spray, and one which I use regularly. It seems to nurture the spirit, at the same time that it is relieving stress from the aura. I use it usually twice a day in the seminar space when I'm teaching, as it helps to remove any build-up of 'leftovers' in the room from people processing the essences. The benefit is always felt immediately by everyone within the space. The beige labelled spray with its Rose Otto oil has a greater impact on the heart chakra than the blue-labelled option. Both have a citrus oil component for cleansing and freshness.

If someone is feeling anxious or upset, this spray would be very helpful. Spray well over the top of the head and let it waft down for best effect.

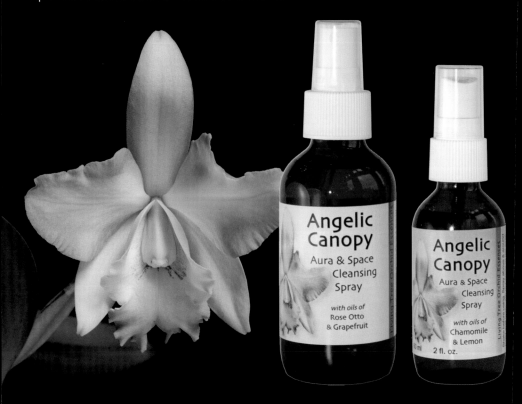

Being Present Aura Spray

Very helpful for adjusting to the local time-zone after long distance air travel (for best results, use as well the Being Present drops, or Being in Time drops). Helps bring one fully to the present after travel of any distance, whether by plane, car, train or boat. We can become a bit 'psychically stretched' over the route of our journey. Being Present Aura Spray addresses this instantly. In the same way, this spray is very helpful at the beginning of nearly any therapeutic session, to help the client be fully present, rather than distracted by the journey they made to reach the therapist. By being more fully present, the healing work of the therapist is then capable of being deeper & more effective. Being Present Aura Spray also helps the therapist to be fully present for the client.

This spray provided me with my most powerful-ever aura spray experience. We had just created it in 2003 when I had to drive from England to Germany. After 10 hours of motorway and autobahn, I arrived at my friend's house. In the first minute after arriving I got out the spray to demonstrate it, and was astonished at the effect. I realized that some part of my psyche had until then been stretched out over the last 100 km of autobahn, and the moment I sprayed myself, I felt my dispersed energy come back to the here and now of my body's immediate space, almost like reeling in a fish. This effect happened though in the space of roughly one second as the spray wafted down over me. One is left feeling more centred, balanced and gently grounded.

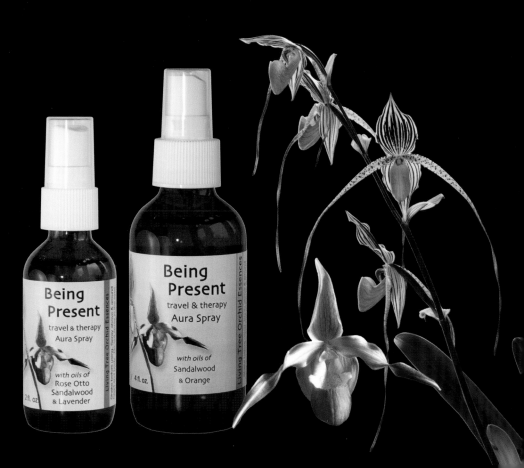

Clearing & Releasing Spray

This spray is to the Angelic Canopy spray what extra strong bleach is to ordinary bleach. When there are particularly challenging situations, perhaps with a karmic element, then this spray is our most powerful clearing and cleansing combination.

Use this spray to help cleanse an aura or a whole building. Use it in a classroom or office at the end of the day, to clear the space for the following day. Therapists would be best to use the Angelic Canopy spray in their treatment room between most clients, but to use the Clearing & Releasing spray at the end of the day, or after an especially difficult client. Sessions with clients are always better if the client is not having to deal with the previous client's energetic 'leftovers'.

Feng Shui practitioners will find that this spray is able to bring about beneficial shifts within challenging spaces. Parents may wish to occasionally spray their teenage children's rooms. Whatever the challenge, this spray is likely to be a great help.

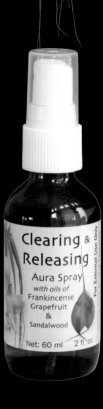
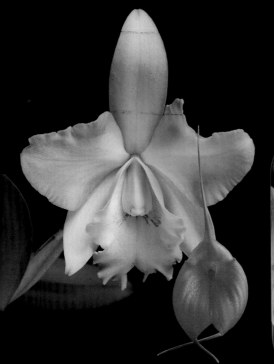
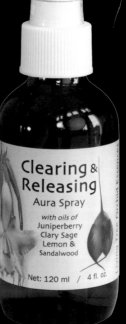

Clearing & Releasing Aura Spray with oils of Juniperberry Clary Sage Lemon & Sandalwood Net: 120 ml / 4 fl. oz.

Clearing & Releasing Aura Spray with oils of Frankincense Grapefruit & Sandalwood Net: 60 ml 2 fl. oz.

Gentle Sleep Aura Spray

Getting a good night's sleep can be a big challenge for many people these days, with a variety of factors conspiring to keep us awake. Gentle Sleep has been created using three of the most calming and relaxing of the orchids (Purity of Heart, Behold the Silence and Boundless Peace), and also the essence of Rhododendron griffithianum, which I made here in Achamore Gardens beside the house.

If the tensions of the day are keeping you wound up, then this spray can help to melt them away. Spray it several times over the top of the head twenty minutes before going to bed, and spray it in the bedroom as well in the same way you would use a space-clearing spray. Use the spray when traveling, for example to help settle and shift the energies of a hotel room. (In the morning and afternoon use the Being Present spray to help get over jetlag.)

The beige-labelled version is more likely to appeal to children, and to those adults who like the rose otto fragrance.

If you are in the UK, then also consider using either the Soul Shield drops or spray, to help address the extra challenge presented by the thousands of Tetra masts all across the country, which are broadcasting a frequency that is the same as our waking-state brainwave pattern. This is in effect a powerful electro-magnetic stimulant, which is preventing millions of people in the UK from getting a decent night's sleep. Take Soul Shield by day, and use Gentle Sleep at night to get the optimum benefit.

88

Positive Flow Aura Spray

Despite my own wonderful experiences of various aura
sprays over the years, I will admit to having been a little bit
surprised by the reports we have had back over the past
year of the efficacy of the Positive Flow spray. My bias
has always been in favour of the drops, thinking that they
must be inherently more powerful. However the
feedback suggests that the spray form of this
combination is every bit as powerful as the drops.

A woman got a good job in the midst of the recession
after several years of being a mum; her husband's
business came back from the brink of liquidation. A
woman in Japan sprayed her husband, whose
company was in trouble for a lack of orders; the same
day he started getting large orders suddenly. Our
distributor in Canada sprayed himself, and 15 minutes
later had a call from a major company he had been
attempting to supply for many months: they simply
wanted to let him know that they were indeed going to
have his company supply them. An actor got further
work confirmed, after using the spray daily for a week.
And a woman in Japan sprayed herself and her purse,
and ended up winning a substantial sum on the
national lottery.

These are just a few of the reports we have had back
from our customers and our distributors. Our own
experience mirrors these stories: we created the
combination in March 2009, and our sales of the
LTOE grew very well last year, despite the global
financial climate. The potency of the spray has
been an eye-opener for me, and marvelous to hear
and experience.

Use the Positive Flow spray regularly in the
home or office, and over yourself, to help bring
the flow of energy you want to see in your life
and work.

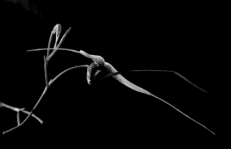
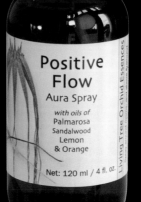
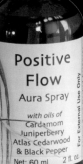

Positive
Flow
Aura Spray

with oils of
Palmarosa
Sandalwood
Lemon
& Orange

Living Tree Orchid Essences

Net: 120 ml / 4 fl. oz.

Positive
Flow
Aura Spray

with oils of
Cardamom
Juniperberry
Atlas Cedarwood
& Black Pepper

Net: 60 ml   2 fl. oz.

For External Use Only

Soul Shield Aura Spray

Provides protection for the body's aura or a living space against the incursion of negative psychic energies.

When I first looked at the combination of these three orchid essences with Peter Tadd, he asked me if we really needed such a high degree of psychic protection, because this one was "like titanium". I explained to him that in all the years of running our business, we had never once have a customer ask us for a "moderate strength" essence for protection, that they always wanted the strongest one we had. "Well then, this is it!" he replied. And over the years since we have indeed found it to be a very powerful combination for precisely that. The name for the combination was Peter's suggestion, and it has always seemed very apt.

Use this spray when traveling into a city for the day, or whenever you may be in large crowded spaces.

Soul Shield spray is also helpful if your work involves sitting in front of computer screens for long hours. Spraying yourself two or three times a week should suffice. Therapists will usually be better off using the Angelic Canopy spray between clients, reserving the use of Soul Shield for themselves primarily when they know they will be seeing a very challenging client. If a client has opened up deeply in a session, they may benefit from being sprayed before leaving the treament room, due to their feeling somewhat vulnerable.

Soul Shield® psychic protection Aura Spray with oils of Grapefruit Sandalwood & Juniperberry Net: 60 ml 2 fl. oz

Soul Shield™ psychic protection Aura Spray with oils of Clary Sage & Lemongrass

Temple of Light Aura Spray

This spray was created to meet an interesting circumstance which Dr. Brito-Babapulle found himself having to address: how to bring about the needed energetic shifts in clients who were unable (for religious or other reasons) to take the Temple of Light combination essence as drops.

As with the drops form this spray was created to meet a specific problem in that there can be an incongruity between the Ba-hui point and the Inner Chamber of the Heart chakra, and the Crown & Heart chakras as well. Real healing is frustrated when these four points are not harmonized. Adrian created this combination several years ago to resolve this incongruity.

In the drop form there are two versions, one with three of the orchids, and the other with five. For the spray form with rose otto as the fragrance, Spirit of the Higher Heart and the 24 karat Gold essences were added in order to achieve the same impact as the drops versions. The alternate in the beige label, with lemon and sandalwood oils, also has the Gold essence, but instead of our Spirit of the Higher Heart, it has the White Orchid (*Cephalanthera longifolia*) essence from the Himalayan Flower Enhancers range included. Through his TEK muscle testing work, Adrian was able to determine that these two formulas had the same impact on the four points of potential incongruity referred to above.

Temple of Light may also be used for space clearing purposes, if Clearing & Releasing or the Angelic Canopy sprays are not to hand.

White Beauty Aura Spray

This was the very first of our aura sprays that we made, and this Spring is its 10th anniversary. From the outset it has always been made with Bulgarian rose otto as its fragrance, though we now also offer it with Sandalwood and Atlas Cedarwood as an alternative.

This spray brings a beautiful energy of unconditional love into the crown chakra and heart centre, and is calming and relaxing. I remember Peter saw a column of white light opening up above the crown chakra of our office manager Margaret Gallier many years ago when White Beauty was sprayed over her. On another occasion SSK was visiting the Living Tree, and I sprayed this over the top of her head, giving the spray pump 7 or 8 'whooshes'... SSK dropped to her knees and melted into the floor in ecstasy. She told me afterwards that this was the single most powerful experience of a flower essence she had ever had.

We once had visitors to our premises in Milland (The Living Tree), who had nearly been in a terrible accident on the motorway on their journey getting to us: a large lorry had almost overturned just in front of them. They were still shaken when they arrived, though an hour and a half had passed since the incident. I gave them both a spray with the White Beauty spray, and I then left them in their camper van outside. A few minutes later they told me that until I had sprayed them, they had not really arrived, that the fright they had received had been pre-occupying them up until that moment of being sprayed. The effect of the White Beauty spray was that of instant relief, their anxiety immediately and quite simply vanishing.

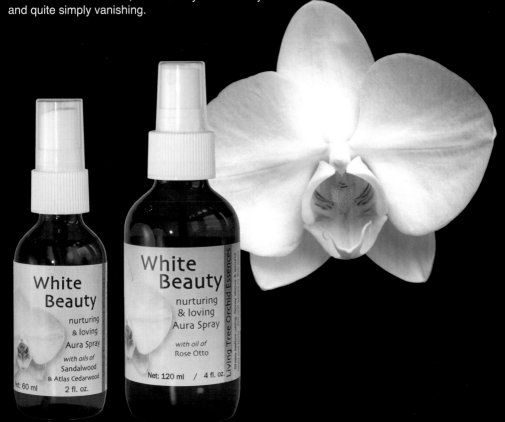

Orchid Greeting Cards
Building bridges
of understanding with family,
friends and colleagues
in a very gentle manner.

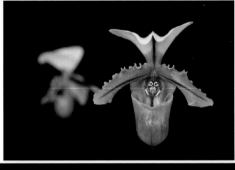

Recently we produced a set of 8 large Greeting Cards, with a selection of my best photos. I see these as serving several purposes, but one of the most important is that of helping to bridge the divide of entrenched viewpoints which users of flower essences can sometimes encounter with family and friends. The cards have only botanical information on each orchid shown, and no reference to the essence made with it. Our web address is given, so if someone who is given the card as a gift wishes to explore the topic of orchid essences, they may do so in their own time. In other words, the cards are not 'preaching' at all, yet allow an entry point for dialogue. They present an open door, yet with no onus on the receiver to go further than simply appreciating the beauty of a given orchid. Over the years I have seen very little in the way of 'bridging materials' produced by the flower essence community, and yet we must reach out to a skeptical world around us, and discuss in rational terms the premises of our field of work.

Bulbophyllum longiflorum
Species of orchid found in the forests of Borneo
and elsewhere in SE Asia from sea level up to 1700m.
There are roughly 1200 species in the genus
found throughout the tropics, but especially in SE Asia.

photo © Don Dennis
Achamore House, Isle of Gigha
Argyll Scotland PA41 7AD

tel. 01 583 505 385
www.HealingOrchids.com

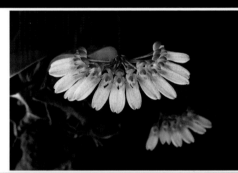

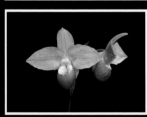
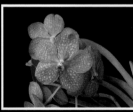
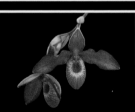

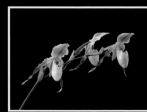
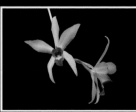
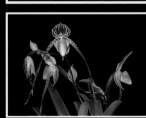

Orchid Photo Cards

This set of photo cards is intended primarily as a tool for helping one to select the most appropriate essence(s) for either yourself or for a friend or client. The best technique is to look at them rapidly one after another, moving through the entire deck, without lingering. It is the immediate visual impact that is the key response. The orchid which grabs your attention will indicate the essence which is likely to be the most suitable one at the moment.

If several cards are chosen, pick the 2 or 3 which created the strongest response.

These cards are the same size as standard playing cards, and fit easily in the hand as well as the handbag.

Our first set of these cards was published in 2007, and so we will be bringing out a supplemental set of cards in 2010 which will include both the newest essences as well as all of our combinations.

My sincere thanks to Junko Terayama, our wonderful Distributor in Japan for the recommendation of this size of card, which has been very popular with our customers. The cards appear to also serve as very good ambassadors for the essences, as they travel around the world.

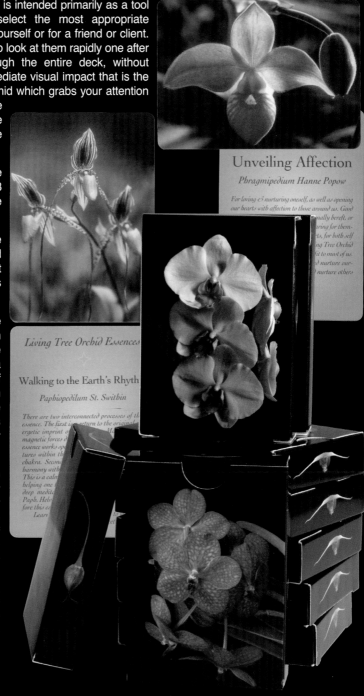

Unveiling Affection

Phragmipedium Hanne Popow

For loving & nurturing oneself, as well as opening our hearts with affection to those around us. Good

Living Tree Orchid Essences

Walking to the Earth's Rhyth

Paphiopedilum St. Swithin

Choosing Essences

There are innumerable ways of selecting essences, either for yourself or for someone else. Here is a list of most of the methods I know of. Anyone of them is likely to be suitable, if it is an approach you feel comfortable with.

1. Reading the information and deciding by reflection on this material.

2. Muscle-testing, also known as Kinesiology.

3. Dowsing, usually with a pendulum.

4. Use the photo cards, by selecting from those photos which most attract your attention.

5. Hold a fingertip over the bottles, and see which one gives a gentle buzz / pull / heat.

Probably the first four of these methods above are the most common in the UK. In general I would recommend a mix of both sides of the brain, as it were: a bit of reasoned knowledge is always useful, especially when used with respect for one's intuition. For example, if a family member is anxious for whatever reason, there is no need to go through a process of intuitive selection using dowsing or muscle-testing, if you know that **Angelic Canopy** is very likely to help straight away. Perhaps these first-aid type uses are easier, insofar as there are a few of the essences which are clearly going to help in most instances. It is when we wish to go deeper in the psyche, to help heal the soul's long-held issues, that the intuitive means of choosing becomes more important.

In general the method I most prefer is the use of photo-cards (like the ones shown on the previous page). This approach has several advantages. First of all, it requires no more than 20 seconds of instruction. It is also at least as accurate as other methods, often astonishingly so. (one example: three generations of women in one family all chose the same card - Just Me - completely independently of one another. This is not a card that is commonly chosen by most people. Yet it spoke directly to a family trait, which was passed from generation to generation.) Furthermore the cards may be used equally well for oneself or for a client or friend, which is exceptional for diagnostic techniques. I like the fact that the image of the orchid is appealing directly to one's intuitive side, readily by-passing the analytical side of the brain, so long as the technique is carried out properly (i.e., by flipping through the cards at a rate of roughly one card per second). Lastly, by printing the cards at the same size as regular playing cards, we have been able to keep the price of the cards very low, making them very affordable.

However, I feel I should mention that my own method is none of the above. Unfortunately I cannot recommend it to others, since I have no idea how it could be taught. I see dots of either blue or white light, which are a kind of yes/no signal from my inner psyche. These began in 1982, after a form of very focused meditation I had devised and briefly tried. I was living on my own for a few months, after I had graduated from university. These dots suddenly made their appearance, and fairly soon I had worked out their pattern of significance. In any case, this is the system I use, which has been very helpful over the years.

Labels & Claims and BAFEP

Flower essence makers have to comply with various regulations, and since the authorities have no simple category for flower essences (unlike say homeopathy, or herbal products), we tend to end up with rather odd things stated on our labels. So for example, we state on our labels that the orchid essences are "dietary supplements" and also ask people to "write for nutritional information". This is because the authorities in the US want to see this on the labels of these odd things that are called "flower essences". Meanwhile the same label actually prevents the essences being imported into Canada, where the government has very different views to their southern neighbour. As for Japan, we have to add 1% salt to the bottles in order for Customs there to let them enter the country.

Another constraint is that in relation to claims. Obviously there are valid reasons of consumer protection, whereby products can only make a "medical claim" if it has a medical license. Fair enough. But this does lead to bizarre aspects of descriptions for all the essence makers. Several of Dr. Bach's remedies address differing aspects of fear. But the authorities in the UK have declared that the word "fear" is a medical term, and so people making Bach Flower Remedies have to instead describe their essences as helping with "fright" - as this is not a medical term.

So you won't find any descriptions of essences helping with depression, since "depression" is a medical term. This is a pity, since any number of essences are able to help in this general area, and some with remarkable effect. So instead we couch our descriptions in vaguely similar wording, such as "helps with when you feel low" or the like. So the reader needs to become adept at reading what is not written, seeing what is implied in many descriptions. And that situation is not likely to change in the foreseeable furture. If we were to go down a legislative route which would allow some degree of medical claims, it would without a doubt bring very expensive licensing with it, which would kill off our industry. And so we put up with what is clearly an unsatisfactory situation.

Nevertheless we are fortunate in the UK to have a very fine organization for flower essence makers, called the British Association of Flower Essence Makers, or BAFEP for short. At AGM's of BAFEP any issues of importance to the membership are discussed, and important developments are relayed via a newsletter and email. It is an organization I can wholly recommend. Further information of course may be found on its website www.BAFEP.com

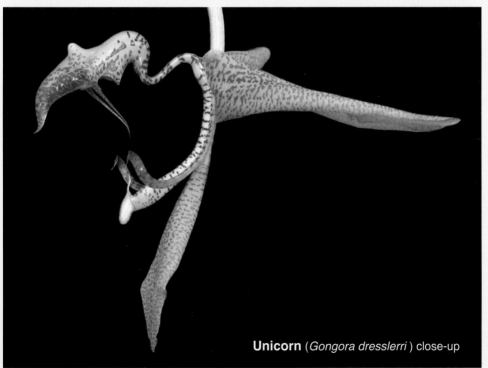

Unicorn (*Gongora dresslerri*) close-up

The Orchid Growers

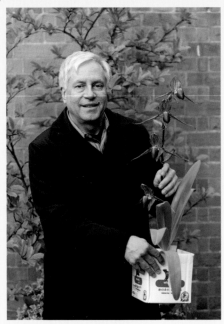

I am often asked where I obtain the orchids we grow in our greenhouses. In fact our work with the essences would be impossible were it not for the network around the world of dedicated commercial and semi-commercial orchid growers. As with essence-making, this is not a line of work one goes into in order to make money. The only possible justification for the endless hours these people devote to the orchids in their care is that it is their passion. Here on these pages I want to give mention to just a few of the people I have been buying orchids from over the past 12 years or so.

Jerry Fischer is the owner of Orchids Limited in Minnesota. I took this photo of him with a *Paph. rothschildianum* by Waddeson Manor in Buckinghamshire, England. Jerry and his wife Yoko have run their business raising and selling orchids for something like 35 years now. He is one of the finest slipper orchid hybridizers in North America, and is also a fount of knowledge about the history of specific plants which have been traded and sold over the past 150 years. It is always a pleasure to talk with Jerry, and to do business with him. Their son Jason looks likely to carry on their business in the decades ahead. One can learn a great deal about orchids and their care by visiting their website www.orchidweb.com.

A very good way to meet orchid growers is to attend orchid shows in your country. Expect to have to travel a bit, but the rewards are great if you do. In early 2008 I traveled to Dresden, Germany to attend a major orchid show there, primarily to collect some orchids from Ecuador I had ordered. Ecuagenera are a very good source of the cloud-forest orchids of Ecuador, and I had dealt with them before very happily.

But a bonus was that I also met a very fine commercial orchid grower from Colombia (Andrea Niessen of Orquideas Del Valle), as well as Günther Ludwig and his wife Inge, who are superb

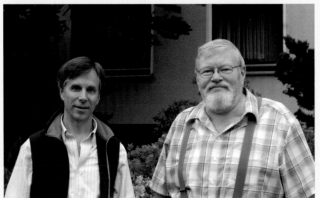

semi-commercial growers near Hanover. I was astonished by the quality of the plants which Günther and Inge had, and bought a number of their orchids. But Günther told me I must visit their home, to see his greenhouse, which I did a few months later.

(Here I am with Günther outside their home in May 2008.)

The sheer quality of the orchids they had at home astonished me. Many of their plants clearly had been carefully tended to for over twenty years. I went home with a good many orchids! Günther reckons he has about 15,000 orchids, and spends about 3 hours a day watering them. A retired engineer, he began growing orchids over 30 years ago. He is now retiring from the orchid growing, as he says it is simply too much work now that he is getting older. As a consequence he is only now selling some plants which for many years he would not have sold, which were part of his personal collection. I mention this to illustrate that it can take some time to meet the various people around your part of the world who may well have orchids that will interest you.

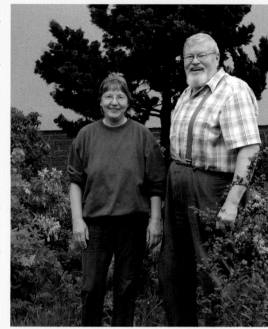

The time and dedication of these growers should not be underestimated; and from where I stand, they are something approaching heroes and heroines, for the years of sacrifice of other pleasures for the sake of these amazing plants of the orchid family.

I have bought orchids from at least a couple of dozen orchid growers over the years. I recommend that you find ones who clearly have a passion for the plants in their care, and who are knowledgable and helpful. And go to the major orchid shows in your region or country. You are not likely to find overseas growers at a county show, but they do take the trouble to travel with their plants (and deal with all the burdensome paperwork) for the major national events. There is a fine one each year in June in Peterborough, England. A marvelous one also takes place each spring in Dresden, Germany. The Botanical Gardens in Glasgow host an orchid show twice a year, on a shoestring budget, but it is well worth attending if you live in Scotland.

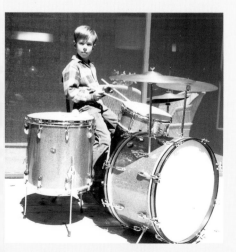

So while it is fine to buy a lovely phalaenopsis orchid at the supermarket, please bear in mind that the supermarket orchids are not even the tip of the iceberg in terms of suggesting the depth and variety of what is to be found in the world of orchids. Get out to a regional orchid show and see for yourself; but beware, you may get bitten by the orchid bug. Current or past interests are no guarantee of immunity! Certainly very few orchid growers have given signs of that predilection in childhood...

Growing Orchids

If you wish to grow orchids, but don't know where to start, then this section is intended for you. If you are already growing orchids within your house but are contemplating expanding past the windowsills, then you may also wish to read further here. But I wish to emphasize that there are many very good books available to help one in some detail, the best of which in my experience being the various titles written by Wilma and Brian Rittershausen, of Burnham Nurseries in England. The Rittershausens have spent decades involved with growing orchids, and write superbly well about a good variety of genera. Their books have both depth and breadth, and with very good photos - always a bonus. Search on the web for their titles, their books will not disappoint.

Perhaps because my first (successfully grown) orchid was a Phragmipedium, I tend to recommend these as an excellent starting point for anyone wishing to grow some orchids. The "phrags" have several merits: (1) it is unlikely that you will ever overwater them; (2) they like any temperature we like indoors, and can generally be grown either cool or warm or inbetween; (3) they have gorgeous, generous blooms which speak readily to us. The only challenging requirement is that you cannot find them in the supermarkets. But let me say a word on that now.

Imagine that you thought the entire world of books was represented by what you could find at the check-out counter of a supermarket. If you then visited a library for the first time, imagine what a shock it would be! In a similar manner, it is highly desirable that you visit a genuine commercial orchid grower at some stage, to view the tremendous variety of what is available today. And that is just the beginning. Web research obviously is a boon to any orchid-lover these days. Visit Jerry Fischer's company's website, www.orchidweb.com. There is a great deal of information about all kinds of different orchids on it, and many thousands of very fine photos to view as well. Another very useful site is www.orchidspecies.com, as well as www.phragweb.info for web browsing.

In order to grow the cloud-forest species (such as the wonderful Scaphosepalums and the gorgeous Masdevallias) you'll need a cool greenhouse, kept above 10 degrees Celsius, and fairly humid. If on the other hand you want to grow the bizarre and exquisite Bulbophyllums, then you'll need a warm greenhouse, kept very humid, and you will need to water them every day for best results. If you want to grow both, you'll need a two-section greenhouse. Ideally there would be a third section, for those orchids that like what are termed "intermediate" temperatures. This becomes increasingly expensive! And yet if you engage in this, then you will be contributing in a small way towards the preservation of orchid species. And that is a very good thing indeed!

The orchids most commonly seen these days are of course the Phalaenopsis, which are also called the Moth orchids, and are seen in supermarkets and shops everywhere. The reason these are so commonly and inexpensively available is because in the early 1960's a Frenchman by the name of LeCoufle discovered it was possible to use a technique known as meristem cloning to bring about mass production of certain types of orchids, the Phalaenopsis being chief amongst these. Using this technique it is literally possible to create a million or ten million identical orchids from a single plant. It is estimated that in 2009 some 200 million Phalaenopsis were sold by the commercial growers in Holland.

This technique is not able to be used with the slipper orchids, and hence their supply is vastly more restricted; this is why you will not find them in the supermarkets.

EM Radiation Challenges

There is little doubt in my mind that one of the greatest health challenges humanity has created for itself is the vast global network of microwave towers and masts for all our new wireless forms of electronic communication. A kind of 'necessary evil' it seems, which we must live with day in and day out whether we wish to or not. That our various governments tolerate this is all the more astonishing given that they know one key fact of microwave radiation: **that its effects on tissue are cumulative**. That is to say, getting a low-level dose over a long period of time has the same effect on our bodies as getting the same amount of radiation at higher intensity over a short period of time. This was discovered in the early 1960's when the military began using microwaves for their major comms links. The engineers performing maintenance on the microwave masts went blind after a few months, as their eyes were being not-so-slowly cooked.

Most of the European countries have fairly strict regulations therefore regarding the levels of microwave radiation that the general population may be exposed to by the various types of equipment around. For example, ships must turn off their radar (which these days is entirely microwave-based) when they are within one kilometre of a port. But in the UK the relevant authorities (the mis-named National Radiological *Protection* Board) have a far more liberal attitude, and state that the only radiation levels which concern them are those high enough to actually increase the temperatures within tissue. This is some 10,000 times higher than the permissible levels of Denmark and Switzerland, for example. Yet in the UK we have an even worse matter to contend with, by far: our national network of Tetra masts.

The danger posed by the cellphone network is minor compared to that represented by Tony Blair's principle domestic technological legacy. Beginning in about 2001, the UK government gave a contract to Airwave, a subsidiary of O2, to install a communications network for the police and emergency services throughout the country. At a cost of over £13 billion Airwave have put up thousands of these Tetra masts across England, Wales and Scotland. The technology used combines microwaves with a very low frequency carrier wave (at 17.65 Hz). The problem with this frequency is that it is in the middle of our waking-state brainwave pattern. When we go to sleep, our brainwaves must get below 3 cycles per second (3 Hz). But the Tetra masts are sending out a high-amplitude wave form which inhibits our ability to get out of the wakened state brain rhythm: it is an electromagnetic equivalent of caffeine.

Not everyone is susceptible to it, just as not everyone is allergic to pollen. But for that large portion of the population who are susceptible to it, this technology is a living nightmare. The lack of sleep is debilitating, leading quite frequently to depression, irritability, anxiety and constant fatigue. It is a blight on the lives of millions of people in the UK today, and has without a doubt led many tens of thousands (at the very least) to an early grave. Pictured here is a Tetra mast above Loch Lomond. If you know someone who is constantly tired, please suggest they look into this topic. They can at least see where their local masts are on this website: www.sitefinder.ofcom.org.uk You should be aware though that this website does not show the masts which are on all Police stations.

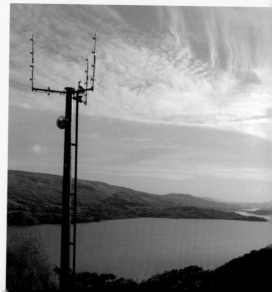

Working with the Living Tree Orchid Essences

What follows here are descriptions from three of the many therapists who work with the Living Tree Orchid Essences. I asked these three both because they are somewhat representative of the broad spectrum of practitioners who use the LTOE, and because they each have a good level of understanding as well as affection for the essences.

Sian Kater has been working in Complementary Medicine in Ayrshire, Scotland for 20 years. She has a background in Therapeutic Massage, Reflexology, Reiki and Classical Homeopathy. Her work involves guiding people towards resolving and healing past hurts and present difficulties while encouraging them to take responsibility for their own process. She draws upon a range of therapeutic techniques, including spiritual counselling, energy medicine, visualization, homeopathic remedies and flower essences. Here is what she has written about her use of the Living Tree Orchid Essences.

Over the years I have suggested essences, books, exercises etc. and occasionally the client would follow through. With the LTOE, however, clients have more often than not had an immediate and beneficial effect from a single dose of an essence I've given them, and so then go away and order what I've suggested.

As well as working with the LTOE on their own, the essences have been an adjunct to everthing I do. Before I did the course I occasionally did guided visualizations; a client was led to the essence of an issue which was then released or healed. This whole process is far quicker with the LTOE. The chosen essence quickly and effortlessly brings up a core issue which is then released either with that one essence or through the use of additional essences. The process is quick, powerful and complete.

Before a Reiki or Reflexology session I get the client to pick a card and then give them a dose of that essence. After the essence the client is generally more centred and receptive and the treatment more powerful as a consequence. Quite a few people, particularly those at the hospice, have had profound spiritual experiences during the session. One cancer patient, who has made remarkable progress with Reiki along with LTOE, had a spontaneous soul retrieval during a treatment last week.

I also often give a LTOE to support clients on a constitutional Homeopathic remedy, when I don't want to intervene and give another remedy too soon.

I can't imagine not using the LTOE in my practice now! Whether the effect is strengthening, centering, cleansing, healing, uplifting or transformative, there is always an effect. Moreover I think my trust and confidence in them is passed on to my clients.

My experiences of the LTOE

Julie Bruton-Seal is a herbalist and essence therapist based near Norfolk, England.

The first time I was at Achamore House I remember being intrigued by the beautiful blue boxes in Don's office. A few days later when Don gave a dose of one of the essences to my friend, I could actually see the energy bubbling around her heart chakra and moving in her body – in fact she said she felt like she was being lifted off the chair. I was impressed as I'd never seen anything like that with any other essences. After learning a bit more about them from Don I went home with a full set of the orchid essences in their beautiful blue boxes, and started using them.

Several years later and I've just upgraded to the even more beautiful purple boxes, which are larger to house the growing range of the essences. In the meantime I had returned to Gigha to attend Don's orchid essence workshop and learn more about the essences, and to meet some of the orchids. Several of the orchids were in full bloom while we were there, and it was a real honour to be with them in person. The most memorable for me was Pushing Back the Night – an enormous flower – and absolutely stunning.

I was really pleased when the photo cards were released, because I find them an ideal way for clients to choose the essences they need. They are nearly always amazed when they turn the cards over after making their selection and see how appropriate the essences they have chosen are for them at that time. I am a herbalist, but I use the orchid cards with most of my clients, and find that I get much better results from the herbs when I give the appropriate orchid essences as well.

I do still use the Australian Bush Flower Essences, and an assortment of other essences, depending on which feel right for a particular client. The orchids are my favourites overall – the plants themselves are such amazing beings, and they seem to have a level of consciousness that is on another level from other plants. In turn the essences seem to go beyond other essences in their sphere of influence.

Personally I found the orchid essences particularly helpful when my father had a stroke and couldn't speak. In the few days before I got there, he was trying really hard to communicate with hand signals but neither my mother nor anyone else there could understand what he was trying so hard to say. He was getting frustrated, and they were at their wits end as to what he trying to tell them. I rang Don for advice and arrived with the recommended essences. Within a few minutes of us taking the essences and sitting quietly together, the non-verbal communication channels were opening and we were able to understand what he had been trying to tell us. One of the remedies for my father was Secret Wisdom, and I think he found it really helpful as he always wanted it when it was offered. He didn't regain the power of speech, but we had some really good 'conversations' with the way smoothed by the essences.

I usually prepare my dosage bottles with distilled aromatic waters instead of the usual brandy and water mixture. Rose and bitter orange blossom are the ones I use most, usually half and half. Elderflower is another I often use – it depends on the individual client and what they need. Sometimes I use rose and bitter orange tinctures as the base, as the alcohol is a preservative. The light floral taste of these works well with the essences.

Orchid Essences and Healing of the Energy Self

Dr. Adrian Brito-Babapulle B.V.SC, B.V.M.S, M.R.C.V.S., M.I.Biol., M.B.S.T.P.,F.R.M.S. originally trained in his native Sri Lanka in Veterinary Medicine, then undertook Pathology training in Glasgow, as well as Microbiology and FRMS (Society of Microscopy). He then trained under Ian Hulme in Applied Kinesiology, and in Homeopathy at the College of Homoeopathy Manchester and the London School of Classical Homoeopathy; he then attended post graduate training with George Vithoulkas. He has now worked for 20 years in Homoeopathy and Applied Kinesiology (Now TEK).

What follows is Adrian's description of the nature of his kinesiological work utilizing the LTOE.

The Healing Centres & Essences

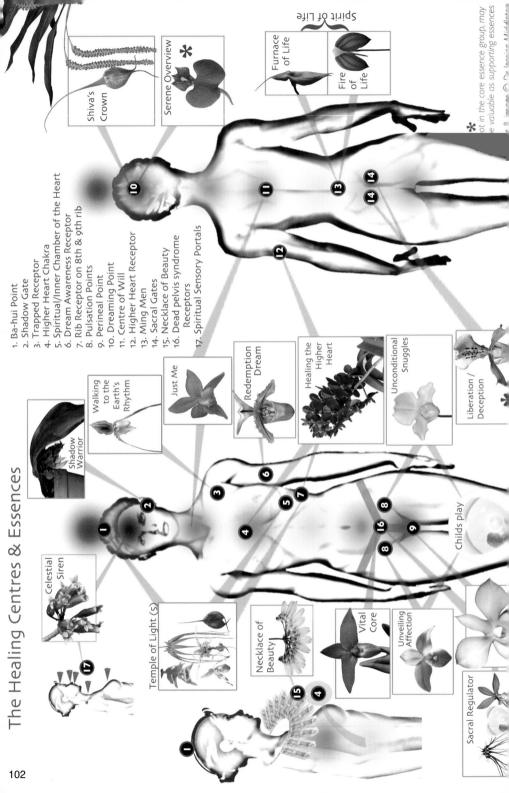

My interest in the power of the orchid essences was born from the observation and correction of energetic points and markers in my patients. Through years of clinical practice I discovered areas of depletion in a persons energy system, which when analysed appropriately, could be corrected with either a homeopathic remedy or an essence. Many of the most effective essences in restoring this balance are orchid essences.

The scope of this document is only a brief description of the testing and therapeutic benefits of the essences, but I have illustrated the important areas below. An assessment of the energy system is done through the use of a modified form of Applied Kinesiology (AK) which I have named **Therapeutic Energy Kinesiology** (TEK). In the description of the techniques I will define any unfamiliar terms when used for the first time.

I see the energy system of the body as multilayered and multifaceted, which some gifted with special senses are able to visualize directly. For those without those particular intuitive abilities the TEK protocol I have devised enables therapists to accurately locate defects in the layers of the energy system, and gives them the appropriate energetic tools to correct such instability. *(Full details about the protocol and how to learn TEK can be obtained from Dr. Jessica Middleton, whose email address is: drjess@mac.com)*

The diagram of the healing centres of the body (see diagram opposite) will give you a feel for the areas in which specific orchid essences interact, and illustrates the layers of the energy system. Many of the orchid essences can produce physical symptoms when consumed as "mother tincture" (the parent essence prior to any dilution). Similar though less striking physical effects can be seen with the "stock" essences (the first level of dilution from the mother tincture – the standard form in which the orchid essences are supplied). These stock essences can be further diluted into dosing bottles as individual or combinations of essences. However In my clinical practice I use only the stock essences, and do not dilute the essences as I cannot predict the effect with prepared dosing bottles. If a combination dosing essence is made for an individual it is beneficial to test this against the patient (using TEK) to check its effect.

In the TEK system we test for emotional, nutritional, physical and energetic imbalances which may be a barrier to healing. Healing is not just the total physical alleviation of symptoms but aims to facilitate the journey of the soul (if you believe in its existence).

In the testing sequence, we can check & correct the important connections within the individual, freeing them from any restraints to the healing process and allowing them to heal at deep levels. It has become more obvious as my work has progressed that a lot of energetic disturbances are in the pelvis, more so in women than in men. If we can correct the energetic blocks to healing in the pelvic energy complex, then a significant degree of healing takes place both physically and energetically.

These blockages often relate to the emotions ANGER, FEAR, GUILT and/or SHAME which affect two gates in the energy system of the pelvis called the "pulsation points" (see diagram opposite). These pelvic points are vital centres of *energetic* communication between people (hence the phrase "we are joined at the hip"). The orchid essences which I have found consistently helpful in correcting these points are **Unveiling Affection** and **Unconditional Snuggles**, along with an essence called **Child's Play**.

Below the pulsation points are a deeper layer of gates which are related to long term energetic or sexual stress. The essences that act at this deeper level are **Sacral Release** (for those withholding their power both sexually & emotionally) and **Vital Core** which brings further energy into this area. **Sacral Release** will bring them the freedom to express themselves if they wish to. **Sacral Regulator** is a new combination which Don and I have recently created, which acts on a gate related to **Sacral Release**, which is the final piece of the puzzle.

During the TEK testing we test for nutritional deficiencies, by using "receptors" which are simply energy gates on the skin often overlying acupuncture meridian points. Unlike meridian points these receptors tend to switch on and off cyclically when working correctly. The nutritional state of the patient can affect the rhythm of the receptors, and is picked up during testing. An example is our test for iron deficiency in which we use the *tensor fascia lata* muscle. This muscle is extremely sensitive to iron loss or transferrin (a protein that binds to iron) deficiency, and correlates well with standard biochemical blood tests for iron. We can temporarily correct the iron deficiency with a homoeopathic potency of iron, which instantly corrects the energetic reading. However long term correction involves the patient supplementing the iron intake until tested again.

Having corrected the nutritional aspect, we then test the energetic centres of the body from the head downwards, using a similar set of receptor gates. These are shown on the diagram on the previous page and correspond to the orchid essences as indicated. These essences have been chosen for repeatability and consistancy of effect in over 95% of patients tested. It is very likely that other essences in the orchid range may have effects as well, which we have as yet not determined.

The range of activity of the chakras is also assessed during TEK. Chakras are energy vortices, which occur at seven points on the body. They usually spin in a clockwise direction when viewed from the front or the back. The chakras have different levels of energetic dominance. The first (base or root) and seventh (crown) chakras lie in the vertical axis and act as axial energetic stabilisers. The fourth (heart) chakra is the governor chakra and is somewhat larger in its presence. The chakras are crucial in establishing the energetic potential of the patient and cure.

Stress is a well known factor which influences the rate of the healing process. It is possible to assess the 6 levels of stress in the body using TEK, which are: Childhood, Adolescence, Current Activity, Need for Control, Over-Controlling and the Fear of Absolute Failure.

The connection between the two halves of the cerebral hemispheres (the right and left sides of the brain) could influence the validity of the testing and so is assessed and corrected if necessary to integrate the energy system.

A series of gates, called portals are seen as " sensory flutes" on the forehead, nose, mouth, throat and heart. These are vulnerable to attack by negative energy, and a key essence in correcting this imbalance is **Celestial Siren**.

At the end of the process we run a check to make sure that the tests and corrections have integrated the entire energy system. After this we can test for the appropriate homeopathic or other therapeutic agent. When the appropriate agent affecting the **whole** organism is chosen using this technique the results border on spectacular. However I would again emphasize that when prescribing an orchid essence to a client, I always use the stock essences, not a dilution from stock. This is because in my experience, the energetic shifts brought about through the TEK process are both more immediate as well as far longer lasting by insisting on the use of the essences at stock strength.

There are numerous other receptors on the body which can be tested by kinesiology e.g. the Weihe points for classical homeopathic remedies, AK receptors for metabolic profiling and the levels of emotional blocks influencing the disease process. We concentrate on the most important of these. Those who are trained kinesiologists will probably have other tests which will be of use. This protocol is for those who are not trained in AK and want a validation of the therapeutic agents they use.

A Few Terms Explained

The **Ba-hui point** is the "place of a hundred gatherings" in Chinese medicine. The Ba-hui point is on the summit of the skull just two finger-widths behind the crown chakra. In the Chinese tradition it governs the major acupuncture meridians.

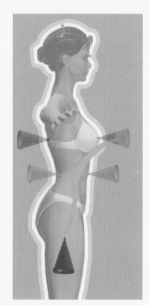

The **Higher Heart centre** can be visualized as a turquoise energy mass above the heart chakra which extends backwards on a 'stalk' into the Spiritual Chamber of the heart and 'roots' downwards into it and through to the 3rd and 1st chakras. (In relation to Spirit of the Higher Heart, this mirrors the shape of the orchid itself in true 'doctrine of signatures'. The roots go down to the root chakra, the body of the plant is in the 3rd chakra, and the blooms act on the Higher Heart chakra.)

The **Ajana centre** is located between the eyebrows, and is distinct from what is traditionally referred to as the "3rd eye" or the 6th chakra. The Ajana centre is a major point of willing things into being. If we have a project, then we will use the Ajana centre (whether knowingly or not) in generating the mental focus to bring it into being. The Ajana centre is not used for clairvoyant seeing - that function is carried out with the 6th chakra/ 3rd eye.

The **Inner Chamber of the Heart** is located just below the heart chakra. It is like the inner temple of the heart, the sacred chamber within the heart.

Adrian's Bibliography

Title	Author	Publisher	ISBN
Sacred Contracts	Carolyn Myss	Bantam	0-553-81494-X
Why People Do Not Heal	Carolyn Myss	Bantam	0-553-50712
Entering the Castle	Mirabai Starr	Free Press	978-0-7432-5532-1
Opening the Energy Gates of Your Body	B. K. Frantzis	North Alantic Books	1-55643-164-3
Physical Examination and Observations in Homeopathy	Filip Degroote		no ISBN
Core Energetics: Developing the Capacity to Love & Heal	Dr John Pierrakos	Life Rhythm	940795000
Nourishing Destiny: The Inner Tradition of Chinese Medicine	Lonny S. Jarrett	Spirit Path Press	966991605
Feng Shui for the Body	Daniel Santos	Quest Books	0-8356-0762-3

A note about the essence called Shadow Facing

This has always been a challenging essence for us. Made with a specie from the South American cloud-forest called *Dracula chimaera*, we have for several years now not included it in our kit, nor described it in our brochures. The principal reason for witholding it in this way is because it *can* help a person to encounter their deepest fears. For this reason we don't wish to have it be at any risk of being used casually or inadvertantly, and so while it is available via our website, we otherwise make the choice not to promote it. I must admit that I feel personally that this is a genus which is best approached with some caution. That Shadow Facing (previously called Sound of Thunder) has value, I am of no doubt. But we simply wish to approach this matter carefully and conscientiously.

Andean Fire   *Resurrecting courage and purpose*   3 drops

Find courage even when overwhelmed by the suffering all around, even in the face of deep physical challenge. Would help those who have been victims of torture or major disasters in this or a past life. This is a major essence to address the horrors of human suffering and a way to experience what is meant by The Compassion of Christ. Helps people of any age to regain the courage which is natural to the soul.

Angelic Canopy   *Balm for the troubled soul*   3 drops

If you can only have one of the Living Tree Orchid Essences, this one should be seriously considered, as it is so helpful in these times. Angelic Canopy brings nurturing to those who are in grief, despair or who have lost hope. Releases the tension from the flight vs. fight response, and helps to strengthen one's alignment to the values of life. "All things can be done in Grace." Very good for space clearing, aura cleansing and for cleansing crystals.

Base Regulator   *Reins in excess libido*   3 drops

Has a powerful effect on the pelvic energy matrix, as well as brings an expansion of conscious awareness around the eyes and head. Reduces excess heat in the liver, and has a cleansing action. Very useful if the person has too powerful a sex drive, with a shift of energy from the pelvic region to higher centres. Then as excess yang sexual energy is reined in, tender intimacy is revealed.

Behold the Silence   *Profound silence, good for meditation*   4 drops

This essence provides a pathway to enter into the profound silence of universal being and invites us into a new relationship with the future. As the reality of the future becomes more and more present in the depth of our inner silence, the past goes back into itself so that we no longer hold the past in the present. In this way our former actions or karmas dissolve. What remains is unobstructed action. Place 4 drops in a small amount of water, and hold in the mouth for 15 seconds to enable the energy to be absorbed through the roof of the mouth and enter the crown chakra. Good for meditation, vision quests, as a preparation for various rituals, and for becoming aware of the sacredness of Nature.

Being in Time   *Be in the local time-zone*   3 drops

Brings the body into nature's local time. Enables therapists to bring the client into contact with the lower half of the body. Helps those who are reluctant to incarnate fully into "the here and now". It does so by harmonising the body's etheric cycles with those same cycles in Nature. In this flow one can manage one's time better, especially when there is the sense of much to do and too little time to do it in. **Great for jet-lag!** The body can immediately harmonise and integrate with the time-zone of the local area.

Being in Grace   *Emotional cleansing*   3 drops

A large and vibrantly purple orchid, the colour of the blooms is central to the action of this essence. This essence brings a cleansing of one's old emotional residue, which has been 'swept under the carpet' of the conscious mind. Its healing process goes deeply into the emotional centre of the brain; it also releases tension from the kidney meridian. Beyond the cleansing this essence helps one step into the inherent dignity and beauty of the healthy, glowing soul.

Boundless Peace   *Gentle relaxed calm*   3 drops
A very relaxing, very 'yin' essence. Experience a sense of buoyancy, floating freedom and ease. Great for relieving tension in the frontal lobes of the brain due to too much mental work. Opens up our psyche to active and productive dreaming. Space takes on a gentle shape with delicate edges. Good for men who may need help in balancing their overly-masculine temperament.

Carnival   *Sensual sheen of the body*   3 drops
Rhythmic and passionately sensual. Very large blooms. Brings an opalescent etheric sheen to the surface of the entire body. Good for those who are too intellectual and live at some distance from their body. Put distance between yourself & the stress of a busy day when you arrive home, and remember to enjoy your wondrous body.

Celestial Siren   *For deep meditation, stillness*   5 drops
The growth habit of this orchid species from SE Asia is remarkable: the long thin pseudobulb hangs down from a branch, held by its roots, and the blooms grow facing down to the earth. Yet the thin tube with nectar at its tip (the "nectary") grows back up towards the sky. And so when we take this essence, there is almost always a pronounced postural change noted: the head tilts forward, and yet there comes a sense of energy moving back up through the head, arcing from the face through the brain and back up out the rear top of the head. This is then followed by a deep, lasting stillness of being. Negative flames of thought are snuffed out like little candles with a snuffer. There is a sense of the Higher Self calling one's soul to remember its deepest and highest potential, to reach towards the inner beauty of enlightenment, yet remaining calm, rooted and centered.

There are in our range several essences (Crown of Consciousness, Secret Wisdom, Behold the Silence, Pushing Back the Night, Guardian of the Inner Journey, Wisdom of Compassion and Serene Overview amongst others) which are deeply appropriate to take whilst meditating. Celestial Siren is also one of these, as it invites a deep inner stillness.

If the vital forces of the body are blocked or low, then it would be good to work also with Vital Core essence, as the physical body needs the energy of its lower chakras working well and harmoniously, for the higher inner journey of spirit to fully unfold.

Clear Mind   *Mentally calm and clear*   5 drops
Clears and calms the mind offering clarity of perception and reflection. Eases mental tension from the mid-brain. "The Mental Break" essence. Think of the clarity of a pale & clear gemstone; the calm of a cool, cloudless, still winter's night. A full moon reflected on a quiet lake. Let your soul listen to the stillness within.

Clearing The Way / Self Belief   *Self-confidence*   3 drops
When self-confidence is needed. This essence strengthens belief in one's own inner and outer spiritual resources, and one's ability to move forward with projects and goals. A wonderful "can do" essence. Also relaxes tension in the 8th chakra, which can result from trying too hard to be in control of everything in our lives.

Core of Being   *Calm yet strong inner alignment*   3 drops

A very important essence to realign to our spiritual axis. This essence enters into one's causal body, which is the "Spiritual White Light". It appears as the central axis, a small-diameter shaft of light running parallel to and just in front of the spine. It is the origin of the chakra system. In a gentle yet profound movement, the essence helps us to align to the higher chakras that compose and create the causal body Light shaft and surrounding causal and celestial auric fields. In doing so, the etheric, astral and mental bodies harmonise very well.

Core Release   *Expansion of intuition*   3 drops

Core release produces an enhanced level of intuition and a 360 degree awareness of one's surroundings. Significant effect on the pelvic centres and on the head, ajna point and crown chakras. Taking the essence creates a wonderful sense of connection to all the energies around us, a profound essence. Resonates with the Liver meridian.

Crown of Consciousness   *Meditate in the Heart of Being*   3 drops

A complete experience of the entire crown chakra. THIS IS A BIG ESSENCE. This essence wishes to welcome you home to the Hall of Records, a space within, where you might find the Living Word of God, the Wisdom of Creation. Surrender to the Beyond that is within and without. Patience. Learn adaptability in approaching the Heart of Mystery, the Light of Consciousness, the Shrine of Shrines.

Direct Vision   *Awakens the 3rd eye*   3 drops

Potentially a powerful awakener of the brow chakra, to be used quite consciously in meditation and vision quests. This is the same orchid that produced New Vitality, but the making of Direct Vision took place six months prior, when the two blooms were facing in the same direction. This alignment imparts a tremendous intensity of the orchid's energy, experienced primarily in the 3rd eye.

Fire of Life   *Revitalized Higher Will*   3 drops

The Fire of Life is the masculine complement to Furnace of of Life. Its yang energy helps the highest of universal energies to incarnate into consciousness, and sets this energy flowing into the centre of one's being. Fire of Life gives courage and purpose to the journey of the soul. It is the Yang energy to the yin energy of Furnace of Life. In observing the bloom of this orchid, it is remarkable how attractive it is to those who feel oppressed, suppressed or unable to express themselves. It breathes new life into the (dwindling) flames of the Ming Men point, thereby strengthening the will of the individual to make choices more in line with highest universal intentions, providing a revitalised opportunity to fulfil ones deepest spiritual destiny.

Furnace of Life   *Rekindle the inner flame*   3 drops

Rekindles the fires of the Kjng Men point. Furnace of Life helps to clear the mist from the lens of perception of the observer, enabling the truth of any given situation to reveal itself effortlessly. Furnace of Life is the female principle, the intention of which is to incarnate our own divine light into consciousness, and to enable us to feel our cosmic purpose. For those whose feminine aspect has been threatened or suppressed, it is best to take Necklace of Beauty first for a few days. Then Furnace of Life will far more readily be able to enter one's chakra system.

Golden Radiance   *Glow with your inner light*   3 drops
To bring one into awareness of the radiance of one's Inner Light, the
"Ground of Being". Golden Radiance honours the spiritual path above all
else. This essence opens the throat chakra and connects to a source of inner
wisdom which appears as golden light within the inner chamber of the heart
chakra. When the inner chamber opens, its "light" can ascend into the throat chakra.
Fundamentally not a remedy, but rather an essence for developing a spiritual perspective of
everyday life. Probably our most universal essence.

Guardian of the Inner Journey   *Look & travel within*   3 drops
Brings the courage to look at the shadows and fears which inhibit progress on one's
spiritual journey. A deeply serious essence, can be taken to enhance meditation.
Paired energetically with Walking to the Earth's Rhythm, which should be taken after
meditating with Guardian of the Inner Journey, for grounding and easing back from
the possible inner intensity which Guardian of the Inner Journey can bring.

Hara to Heart   *Be grounded before going higher*   3 drops
Very good for people who are reluctant to incarnate. This essence brings energy down
to the 2nd chakra (Hara), then up through the solar plexus and into the heart chakra.
Helps eliminate conflicting emotions. Helps one to be incarnate with a sense of purpose.
This essence infuses the halo with a diamond-like appearance, indicating higher
chakra activity. NB. Take this essence 2 or 3 times within a 10 minute period for
best effect and wait for one to three days before repeating or use it as a one off.

Healing the Higher Heart   *Key for a healthy heart chakra*   5 drops
The one orchid produced two forms, two essences: one by itself
(Spirit of the Higher Heart) and this one which has essence of 24
karat gold added, which enhances the orchid's energetic action. The
higher heart chakra is a light turquoise color and is responsible for
releasing the heart chakra from emotional blocks (either karmic or
current). This essence centers itself in the spiritual chamber of the
heart and sends it roots into the 3rd & root chakras. It then enters &
heals the higher heart chakra.

Heart of Light   *Removes emotional armour, brings insight*   3 drops
Heart of Light provides a liberating feeling as it launches our emotional body
out of old patterns of defensiveness into Universal Connectedness to be
experienced an on-going pattern of endless flow. Rapidly releases emotional
armouring of the heart, expanding the chest, allowing the heart chakra to
extend back and re-connect to the central axis of the aura. The 12th chakra
then awakens our memory of our unique spiritual inception into the
Time/Space continuum. The 15th chakra opens as well to the residence of
"Universal Order", the home of sacred geometry.
This essence was made with the same hybrid used to make Messenger of
the Heart. Different plants were used for each essence, & the two
essences were made a few years apart from each other. And while
there are some connections we see between the two, the differences
are considerable.

Internal Cleansing   *For a healthy digestive tract*   4 drops
This essence helps the internal cleansing of the body. Working away without fanfare, it helps to clear up our etheric body's 'residuals' - little packets of leftovers. Acts on the energetic pathways of the throat, stomach, large intestines and liver, assisting with detoxification. Wrapped in foil when in the kit, as it is energetically very different from the other essences in the line.

Joyous Purification   *Retrieve purity of the root chakra*   5 drops
Purifying the base chakra for both men and women. For men it can initiate them into the feminine understanding of purity and innocence. Whereas we often think of purification as a painful or arduous process, the action of this essence results in an experience of joy. For women it will help with certain sexual abuse issues by re-establishing the natural innocence of the root chakra in a natural rise of white etheric light. This light moves very easily and effectively, allowing one to work therapeutically with the issues that have been held subconsciously in the root chakra.

Just Me   *It's just fine being me!*   3 drops
Celebrate one's unique personality without being influenced by projections and expectations of others. Accept our limitations not as negative identities but as momentary states of our development on the journey of individuation. The world is in need of more characters. Very good for children who have do not feel loved, or who feel misunderstood.

Knight's Cloak   *A major protection essence*   3 drops
In dark times it may well be prudent to cloak one's light, to enable one to carry the knowledge of inner truth without risk of drawing the attention of negative forces. This essence provides protection to help one to remain concealed from those who may threaten, bringing a sense of both invisibility and invincibility. Strengthens and protects the back of the throat chakra, which is the area of first vulnerability in psychic attacks. **Knight's Cloak** is one of three elements of the combination **Soul Shield**.

Laughing Butterflies   *Dance with playful joy*   3 drops
This essence is very playful, very forgiving, a large belly laugh from the happy Buddha. Leave your troubles behind, effortlessly and smoothly swirling away. Good for anyone who is prone to take themselves too seriously or for those who feel emotionally stuck. **Laughing Butterflies** enters the solar plexus like two people dancing together in perfect harmony. Think of Ginger Rogers and Fred Astaire spiralling across the floor in each other's arms. Helps the brow and throat chakras, as well as the eyes.

Liberation/Deception   *Think and reflect with deep clarity*   3 drops
How do we fool ourselves by projecting what we desire and not truly need? When is the "light" just a diversion? What is true liberation? Is it to be found in political expression or smoking dope or trance dancing? Even on the inner path, how can we fool ourselves in the quest for freedom? Where do we find the Buddha sitting? This essence operates at two main levels. At the more obvious level, it provides endurance and 'upward' strength, as well as helping to cleanse, strengthen and protect the aura. It would help with any new venture as well. Also about recognising & accepting inner beauty.

Life Direction (Lanata)   *Step back to look ahead*   3 drops
Picture the drawing of a bowstring to establish the direction of an
arrow's flight. So it is in our lives that our goals and our life's direction is best achieved by
stepping back deeply within ourselves. The hand pulls back and we make contact with the
centre of the chest, the heart. Being centred in this way ensures our best aim and direction.
Activates the heart and throat chakras.

Light of My Eye   *Helps us to see more clearly*   4 drops
Frog looks up to the stars and Great Spirit replies showering light from the heavens.
Frogs are able to literally see starlight and register this light one photon at a time
on the retina. In a similar fashion, this essence wants to help us 'see
beyond the veil'. Helps bring etheric light into one's eyes even in dark
times, such as in winter. (See also **Mercutio**, and **Laughing Butterflies**.) In
native cultures the eagle represents the power of, Great Spirit. It is swift and
sure in its flight and the model of spiritual power. Full of starlight froggy jumps off
of his pad and plunges into life and the world of water.

Mercutio   *Enjoy the dance of words*   3 drops
Poise, humour and verbal repartee are the hallmarks of
Mercutio, the marvelous character in Romeo and Juliet.
Enjoy the movement of words and meaning. Also good
for those who are taking things (or themselves) too
seriously; good for students who are being bullied. Stand back from the drama, get the
overview, like the director of a play and watch the interplay between actors and dialogue.
Brings white etheric light into the eyes, so this essence is recommended if one has been
reading a great deal. (See also **Light of My Eye,** and **Laughing Butterflies.**)

Messenger of the Heart   *Give voice to your feelings*   3 drops
Give voice to the heart and communicate what you are feeling, without
fear of the consequences for speaking your truth. To help become more
aware of what is deeply valued within the heart. Picture a messenger on
a white horse, galloping along in your heart spirited by the desire to be true,
and to speak and convey what is honest and true in your heart.

Necklace of Beauty   *Experience the beauty within*   3 drops
brings an exquisite, beautiful and loving energy to the area above
the higher heart chakra but below the throat chakra, enabling one
to feel uplifted, loved and at peace. This essence honours one's
inner beauty, and the light of one's true being. Also enables the ego
or shadow side to ease its hold, so the soul can continue its journey
into light. Necklace of Beauty appears to 'open the gate' for one to experience
more fully the high consciousness of the combination Spirit of Life (or its two components
Fire of Life and Furnace of Life).

New Vitality   *Boost your stamina*   3 drops
The plant from which this essence was made very clearly indicates its
gift of stamina in that the blooms come in succession on each 'spike', and
each given spike of the plant can be in bloom for a year or more. Provides
vitality under circumstances of long-standing tiredness and exhaustion. This
essence can give an energy boost to see one through such difficult periods.

Positive Outcome   *Helps cultivate a positive frame of mind*   3 drops
Maintains undeterred optimism accompanied by remarkable stamina. With
this essence the goal of any project is never out of sight, "like a pole-
vaulter visualizing going over the bar before the run up to the big leap."
Use this essence to experience being drawn ever forwards.   Discover how
to remain positive and steadfast to your own rainbow's end.

Protective Presence   *A bodyguard from the devic realm*   3 drops
This essence is good for people who are travelling to places where personal safety
is challenged. Useful in times of major change (such as moving house
or career changes) to provide continuity and protection. It helps one to
re-connect with inner strength. This orchid bears a resemblance to the
protective "wrathful deities" of Tibetan Buddhism with the sense that a spiritual
presence says "I go before you". Can aid in discovering that actual protection
comes from realizing the true nature of Being, which we find deep within.

Purity of Heart   *Slow down, take your time*   3 drops
Useful for the stress of feeling there is not enough time. Like the slow,
clear,   well-spaced tones of a sitar, this essence conveys the
understanding that there is "enough time to do anything".
Epitomises the Kaffa type of the Indian Ayurvedic system, which is
slow and unhurried, never compelled to rush. Brings white light to the
upper heart chakra, the brow and sacral chakras, and into the blood.

Pushing Back the Night   *Building the inner Temple*   4 drops
Produces a state of mind where vision and light become inseparable. Helps
elevate our thoughts to the point where we can see the Sacred in life. An
essence to help heal the destiny of humanity. Not only does it aid our own
personal growth, but also invites the Light of the Future to Take Back the
Night. Blockages in the bahui centre, the Chinese Crown Chakra point, (on
the top of the head) are pushed out of the auric field; and in doing so, this
enables us to extend an awareness vertically into a temple within a celestial
domain. In this way the microcosm affects the macrocosm. In this time when
many negative karmas are being released upon the world, this essence is
especially important for helping people not to be distracted from a spiritual
purpose and light.

Redemption Dream   *Resolving & healing guilt & shame*   3 drops
Redemption Dream helps the psyche to address deep layers of guilt or
shame, through bringing a shift to our dreams, enabling the mind to either
consciously or unconsciously to resolve these issues. Guilt and shame are likely to cause a
kind of compression (or suppression) of the heart chakra, particularly by means of blocking
the higher heart chakra's ability to cleanse and heal the heart chakra.
Through this blocking of the heart's energy, we lose the ability to love
unconditionally, and thereby also lose inner peace. In this way one can see
how guilt or shame can be major hindrances of our spiritual path.

Redemption Dream helps us to remove these hindrances of the heart,
specifically through vivifying and re-integrating our dreams at night, to
allow ancient and deeply held issues to be aired as it were in the Theatre
of the Psyche. In general, most people will benefit from taking Redemption

Dream in the days before taking Necklace of Beauty; or at the very least, the exquisite energy of the latter will be more readily accessed and fully felt if Redemption Dream has been worked with first.

Releasing Karmic Patterns   *Let go of old deep patterns & beliefs*   3 drops
Releases karmic patterns which are held in the eighth chakra. The eighth chakra indicates how spiritual knowledge & power have been misused in the past. This essence can make us feel like we are spiralling out into the cosmos, thus it can feel intimidating due to the feeling of being taken up and away. Helps free up rigid belief patterns or merely parroted ideas held in the eighth chakra . Helps us use and choose words wisely when we speak.

Renewing Life   *Bring etheric health to the cellular level*   3 drops
A very gentle, quiet essence, yet profound in its ability to reach many levels at once. Clears ancient negative energetic patterns at the cellular level via the 1st, 8th, 10th and 12th chakras, renewing one's inherent health. The root chakra governs cellular patterning and when combined with the higher chakra action of the 10th chakra (the Source of White Light) and the 12th chakra (the wholeness of the universe), it makes this essence a strong candidate for healing at that level.   Very helpful when added to skin creams.

Rising to the Call of Beauty   *Beauty is truth, truth beauty*   4 drops
This essence is about aligning & identifying with beauty. As modern societies have distanced themselves from natural beauty and inner beauty, dissonance, distortion and self- degradation have followed. This has influenced us in ways that distract us from the simple beauty in nature and in ourselves. What are the innate properties of beauty? Proportion, integrity, harmony and respect for the forces and mathematical dimensions found in sacred geometry. When beauty is a guide, the results of our actions naturally and harmoniously follow Universal Principles. Beauty's strength will banish evil and ugliness from her presence. Helpful in relieving shoulder tension at the end of a working day.

Sacral Release   *For pelvic health at the etheric level*   3 drops
Sacral Release provides vital energy to help with the release process and breaks a vicious cycle of low energy and low achievement. It helps to ground and release tensions stemming from subconscious patterns held in the 2nd chakra, which drop down to the earth. The energy in this essence affirms you are safe, strong and healthy.

Secret Wisdom   *Profound stillness in meditation*   3 drops
"Secret Wisdom" returns our focus into the depth to the Inner Divine that is found in the Inner Chamber of the Heart Chakra, which lies just beneath the heart chakra. From here a vision arises, the embodiment of serenity and silence which activates the chakras in the head, and then directly awakens the 11th chakra.   This transcendental chakra offers us the perception based on compassion and wisdom that honours "self as other and other as self" and that "life is essentially a mirror of our own thoughts and actions". This essence is recommended for those who are well on their way along the spiritual path.

Serendipity   *Leap out of the rut, with new insights*   3 drops
Very helpful when one is bogged down with too many responsibilities or just feeling stuck. Move into action with deeper dimensions of one's being. An effective antidote to being stuck in a rut. Helps bring new insights into meditation.

Serene Overview (Devata)   *View the landscape of your life*   3 drops
Creates the space within you for a serene overview and perspective on your life. Devata refers to the spiritual potential of the soul, to the human heart warming the world with its noble presence. This spiritual charisma can be found in our nobler qualities: quietly regal, insistent but not aggressive, acting with integrity. A deep honouring of the mature feminine aspect of the soul. "Beauty is Inner Truth made Perfect".

Settling with a Smile   *Good for the digestion*   3 drops
Creates a calm and quiet joy. Helps the energetic lining of the stomach, and the etheric activity of the liver and gall bladder. Good to take after festive indulgences. Helps with emotional upset, giving one a sense of security. When children are studying, this essence will help to maintain focus.

Shadow Warrior   *Keep the shadow side in check*   3 drops
An extraordinary orchid, this essence was brought into being to assist the integration of one's shadow side with the onward journey of the soul into the light. It stops the shadow from interacting negatively with challenging archetypes, and enables grounding of primitive fears. Enters the base of the skull and goes down the causal body to the root chakra and below, connecting the soul to the root of the soul's journey. This essence clears one's inner vision causing a change in perception, a deeper reality, and enhances clairaudience. Shadow Warrior is a very 'yang' essence, and the effect is sustained with a minimum dose.

Shiva's Trident   *Aligning to our spiritual purpose*   3 drops
This essence opens the yang polarity of the meridian system, the baihui point on the top of the head, bringing in a spiralling, very active energy. This essence is to a large degree the masculine counterpart to Serene Overview, where we go inside to rediscover the Divine. Here the realignment to our spiritual purpose found at the outermost level of the universe opens the wisdom aspect of the crown chakra.

Songline   *Attune to your unique inner path*   3 drops
To help one attune to one's unique spiritual path, that path which is yours and yours alone. How many steps forward on that path do we take in a lifetime? How easily we become distracted from our deep inner path. Songline conveys a song of Love. By helping to re-establish the halo of light over the crown chakra, it awakens one to the responsibility of sound & speech and assists in being true to oneself - an attunement to deep vows. Connects one as well to the sounds & choirs of the angelic realm.

Source of Life   *Cleansing & balancing the pelvic energies*   5 drops
Acts on the pelvic pulsation points, and has its strongest action on the perineum, cleansing & revitalizing it. Clears ancestral memories held in the 1st & 2nd chakras.

Spirit of the Higher Heart   5 drops
The best follow-on for Healing the Higher Heart
The higher heart chakra is above the heart chakra and has a root into the
spiritual chamber of the heart. The higher heart chakra is a light turquoise
color and is responsible for releasing the heart chakra from emotional blocks
(either karmic or current). This essence centers itself in the spiritual chamber of
the heart and sends it roots into the 3rd & root chakras. It enters & warms the higher
heart chakra freeing you to appreciate Love.

Totem   *Connecting with your animal spirit guide*   3 drops
Within the circle there is boundless strength, knowledge, and affirmation of the
goodness that lies at the Heart of Mother Earth and Father Sky. We can
with confidence call upon and /or discover our Power Animals when using
this essence with the clarity, strength & stillness of the timeless heart. This
essence helps us to step into the Hoop of all Nations – the Nations of
Animals, of Peoples, of Galaxies.

Unconditional Snuggles   *Cuddles in a bottle*   3 drops
A gentle, comforting, lasting embrace. Great for adults at the end of a tough
day. Good for children at any time, and especially if waking with night fears.
For children can be combined well with **White Beauty** to give them
reassurance that they are fully loved.

Unicorn   *Focused action*   4 drops
Take a focused, committed and unfailing action. Meet that outer threat
not with aggression but with the clarity of a positive outcome. Highly
recommended for emergencies, major crisises or when one is truely
threatened. This essence helps us to avoid distraction & giving our power
away to a source of potential harm. Clears the energetic pathways of the head
& into the brain by opening the Da-zhui point on the 7th cervical vertebra.

Unveiling Affection   *Opening the heart & loving yourself*   3 drops
For loving & nurturing oneself, as well as opening our hearts with affection
to those around us. Good for anyone who has ever felt emotionally bereft,
or who has difficulty valuing & caring for themselves. To hold affection in our
hearts for both ourselves & others. The first of the LTOE range remains a favorite.

Vital Core   *Energizing the lower chakras & gall bladder meridian*   3 drops
Vital Core is strongly energizing of the Root and 2nd chakras, as well as the gall
bladder meridian. While having some activity on the Crown, Throat and Heart
chakras, its action is primarily in the two lower chakras whereby it provides a
strong 'get up & go' effect. The effect on the 2nd chakra is intriguing:
though energizing, it is not a sexual energizing. It helps to release
stored / blocked energies, including stored negative energies, and
thereby helps to resolve shadow aspects of the Sacral chakra. In
this way, it seeks to restore the natural sacredness of the 2nd chakra.

Phragmipedium besseae is a species of slipper orchid which was
discovered in Peru in 1981. In our process of making this essence, the
orchid requested to have the process take place largely in the evening

and into the dark of the night. A full moon on that clear night shone through the partially-curtained window, its beam upon the orchid and the bowl of water. This not only brought out the yang qualities of the orchid, but also enabled it to better access the shadow aspects of our lower chakras. (This also accounts for Vital Core having some very different qualities to the essence Radiant Strength of the Dancing Light Orchid Essences of the USA, which was made with the same species of slipper orchid.)

Walking to the Earth's Rhythm   *Gently, calmly grounding*   3 drops
There are two interconnected processes of this essence. The first is a return to the original energetic imprint of our DNA. Many electro-magnetic forces disturb this etheric fabric. This essence works specifically to repair very old ruptures within the etheric matrix of the throat chakra. In step two, we find that we are walking in harmony with the rhythm of the Earth herself. This is a calming, soothing and gently grounding essence, good for helping one to gently come back to earth after deep meditations. Learn how to walk, and where to walk by 'listening with the feet'.

White Beauty   *Unconditional love*   5 drops
Envelopes one's aura with unconditional love, akin to that of a mother for a newborn child. Nurturing and de-stressing. Refreshing and mildly relaxing. Can be used as a post-trauma spray for both people & animals. Combine with **Unconditional Snuggles** to help with children's night-fears.

Winged Gold   *The imagination resonating with the soul's destiny*   3 drops
An ancient Chinese gong sounds its tone, awakening one to the inner calling to the fire of the soul's mission and destiny. The weaving of the tapestry of our myriad lives is completed in the utter gracefulness of the dance of the soul which knows its wholeness. Meditate on the peace of this essence to discover the fecundity of the sacred & the flowing purpose of our lives. This essence is very helpful for creative writing.

The Wisdom of Compassion   *In the heart of the Compassionate One*   3 drops
This orchid called out gently and clearly for an essence to be made, with its message of compassion for all beings. Made on the full moon anniversary of the Buddha's enlightenment. The need for this energy is fully apparent in the world at this time. The path of this essence may follow this sequence: It enters the ajana centre, a small but intense point between the brows, a major point of spiritual manifestation. Then it begins encircling the head with a protective energy to finally enter the crown chakra. Its golden light then enters the heart chakra. In meditation this essence is able to reach deeply into the heart chakra, with its transformative effect bringing feelings of joy and optimism, and compassion for all beings.

A Few Words about the Higher Chakras

In the first several years of the making of the essences, our exploration of their qualities had two main routes. The first was our own meditational experiences of the mother tinctures, which is still one of our primary routes to this day. The other was in the discussions with Peter Tadd in relation to his clairvoyant readings of the essences. In that period we didn't have many therapists using the LTOE, and so the information which Peter provided gave a short-cut insight into each essence and its uses. I myself am given to metaphysical reflection on the nature of the Universe and Being, and so is Peter. These discussions about the higher chakras served to give me a deep respect for the orchids themselves; and the orchids became the central focus of our dialogue regarding the higher energetic structure of our existence.

Peter is able to see the chakras within our bodies, as well as the ones above. For him this is a simple reality, akin to the way I see rainbows or sunsets. One of the distinguishing features of orchid essences is that they have an impact on these higher chakras, whereas non-orchid essences for the most part do not. So it was natural for Peter to examine the action of the LTOE into these chakras when doing his clairvoyant readings. I would add that like most people, I certainly do not see chakras at all, higher or lower. Yet I have had very clear experiences over the years of the in-the-body chakras which have led me to know that they certainly exist. In a similar way, I know that there is substantive reality to these higher chakras too.

In the past six years as more and more complimentary health practitioners have been working with the essences, our focus has become more concerned with providing information which is more readily useful to therapists. It isn't easy to bring the higher chakra information into the treatment room, yet I feel there is a valid point in having some delineation and discussion of the higher chakras, almost in the same way that I feel that poetry has an important role in our lives: it can serve to inspire. Peter is currently writing a book on the topic, and anyone wishing to explore this subject further is likely to find it very interesting reading. Visit his website www.petertadd.com to check progress. What follows below are introductory remarks from him regarding the essences & the higher chakras.

One of my first experiences of orchid essences were those made by SSK, with her Dancing Light Orchid essences. This goes back more than a decade, and at the time I felt that they were not for general consumption, as they were so refined & calibrated to higher aspects of our spiritual nature. That was then and now it is very clear that orchids for that very reason are very much part of the Great Paradigm Shift. My work with the LTOE gave me a great appreciation for just how orchids could be so amazing. Prior to examining them I had many experiences with what are called transcendental or cosmic chakras, which are groups of chakras that stack above the crown. There is a set of seven then another set of five; they continue to climb in to double digit numbers. One time I heard the HH Dalai Lama giving a teaching in London, and clairvoyantly saw that he was manifesting the 64th chakra level.

What the higher or cosmic chakras indicate is our level of spiritual development and our ability to be one with life. Here is one way to approach an inquiry into the connection of orchids to the Cosmos: most of the LTOE have been made over a 24 hour period, which at first was a shock to Don and me as this "violated" the classical protocol of making essences in sunlight. This began with the very first of the LTOE, the essence called Unveiling Affection. Indeed some have been made only at night. But the orchids are able to use light from other suns which we call stars. We forget that we are influenced by the planets in our solar system and the constellations of stars. We over-identify with being human or British or Brazilian or whatever as we get on with our daily tasks that we forget our spirituality, our higher nature. We are each one of us part of the Great Mystery. The orchids use starlight and cosmic energy seen as pure white & calm light, which in sanskrit is called sattva. This pure pristine consciousness reflects the very structure and qualities of our own cosmic chakras; in Chinese qi gong this is called original qi or shen and which Buddhists call bodhicitta awakened mind, original view.

Orchids are here to bring us back into an alignment with this primal or original Self. They are able to experience Oneness and at the same time distinguish the multiplicity of that singularity, just as the trillions of stars in the heavens are unique yet basically composed of the same and simplest of all elements. Our higher nature appears as a star over us, that my guidance calls an Infinite Point, which is composed of cosmic chakras. There are then chakras that continue to expand outwards beyond that Point into this and other universes.This can be difficult to comprehend mentally, rationally. This is not so different from some of the challenges presented by advanced physics. What David Bohm called the Implicate Order becomes explicit in nature as orchids and orchid essences, and in ourselves as the cosmic chakras.

So lesson one is that orchid essences are here to help us reconnect to our cosmic or transcendental spiritual essence, which is a very pure state of consciousness.

Lesson two is about power as seen in it's purest and highest form. We need to take a huge leap beyond conventional ideas about ourselves and life. Orchids are such refined life forms, and are so unique and unusual that we used to joke that they must have come from the stars. At first encounter I felt most of us were not ready to experience the levels of consciousness embodied by the orchids, and offered via the essences. But life and the world is accelerating and the time has come for those willing (and courageous enough) to embrace the deeper reality these beings present to us. Orchid essences are certainly one way to wake us up. May we all become as powerful, free, beautiful and blissful as our orchid friends.

I want to mention that when I first met Heather Decam I was impressed by her aura. She has a white sphere of refined spiritual energy surrounding her "human aura". This indicates someone who has higher chakras that are very active. On a few occasions I witnessed her essence-making with Don (with whom she has a very old soul-connection) and her ability to invite the Devic levels of the orchids. Heather has one of the most refined clairvoyant gifts.

- Peter Tadd, March 2010

Orchid Conservation

Orchids and their habitats are endangered all over the world is the simple truth of the matter. Tigers and pandas and dolphins naturally grab the headlines, but orchids are every bit as threatened as the great cats. In the past year we learnt of a non-profit organization called the

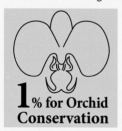

Orchid Conservation Coalition, which is encouraging a marvelous idea. It is asking companies and corporations to donate one percent or more of their net revenue to projects actively involved with in-situ orchid conservation anywhere in the world. The OCC is a grassroots organization of orchid enthusiasts, orchid societies, and orchid businesses run by volunteers.

IFER has now signed up to this program, and this year we are making our first (albeit small!) donation to the Gurukula Botanical Sanctuary in Kerala, India. Now in its 30th year, the GBS is the premier centre for native orchid conservation in the sub-continent. A small yet very dedicated team look after the sanctuary, and appear to have made the GBS their life's work. This is orchid conservation at its finest, and the GBS is well worth a visit. We have links to the GBS and the OCC on our website, and I would highly recommend downloading the pdf about the GBS which is found on our orchid conservation page.

Tropical vs. Native

The orchids we work with have been exclusively tropical ones, and I have no good rational explanation as to why I have not found myself equally interested in the native orchids of the UK or Scotland. I know that in part it has to do with the tropical orchids grabbing my attention first. Slowly, I have been gaining more understanding of the native orchids. In the UK there are just 56 species, and within Scotland as a whole only 26. One may find eleven species on Gigha itself, such as this beautiful species of *Dactylorhiza* which I photographed one June here. I have not yet been drawn to make an essence with any of them; maybe in time it will come, I have no idea.

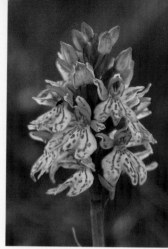

Perhaps it is the sheer richness of opportunity that tropical orchids present, which is so deeply alluring to me. Just within the genus Paphiopedilum, there are more species than are to be found in the whole of northern Europe. So it is a bit like choosing between a library with 26 titles, or one which holds 400,000 titles. Yet it is always good to learn about one's local flora, and I am certainly intending to get to know our local orchids better.

Living Isle Flower Essences (L.I.F.E.)

What has attracted my attention since moving up here to Gigha are the extraordinary blooms to be found in Achamore Gardens. Col. Sir James Horlick was as enamoured of rhododendrons & azaleas as I am of orchids, and to see the gardens in their peak - usually these days in May - is to see rapturous and overwhelming beauty. Succumbing to this, I made several flower essences with rhododendrons one Spring, just two of which we have decided to release at this point: *Rh. griffithianum*, and *Rh. Brocade Plus*.

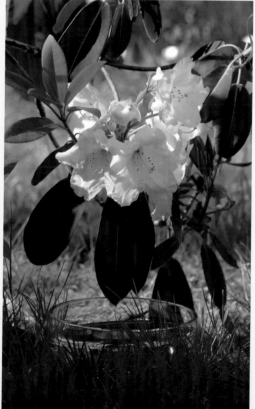

As with the orchids, a non-cutting method was employed. I can see little reason to cut blooms for essence-making unless there is no alternative. Within the confines of Achamore Gardens, I found it fairly easy to be resourceful enough with blooms and bowls to be able to entirely avoid cutting any flowers. Occasionally with a rather high branch I would support the bowl on a tall stool. But many of the rhododendrons have branches trailing near to the ground, so the bowl could be placed just under the blooms on the grass as seen in the photo here. This was the essence of *Rh. griffithianum* in the making; the bowl of water was left under the blooms for about 5 hours, then water was poured over the blooms back into the bowl. A weekday, and a quiet part of the garden is chosen, to avoid disturbance by visitors.

Rhododendron griffithianum

This essence was made with a specie originally found in Sikkim and other parts of the Himalaya. Stunningly beautiful, with nearly all-white blooms (as seen opposite), there are a number of specimen plants found in Achamore Gardens. We found the essence to be very calming and relaxing, and in fact our 'nickname' for the essence was "Peaceful Chill-out". This is not an essence to take at the office when you have a lot of work to get done! But it is wonderful to take to have a relaxing shift of energy into calmness. Many of our customers have encountered it as a component of the combination **Gentle Sleep**, as its yin characteristics complimented the three orchid essences which are found in **Gentle Geisha** and **Gentle Sleep**. This rhododendron essence would be a very good one to bring into a full-body massage treatment, as the client would be helped to relax much more quickly and deeply.

Rhododendron Brocade Plus

Col. Horlick was a keen rhododendron hybridizer, but often neglected to register his resulting crosses. Rh. Brocade Plus is one such hybrid, now in effect part of what is referred to as the "Brocade Group". This was in magnificent bloom when I made the essence with it. There are several specimens in the gardens here, and the one I chose was tucked away in a corner well away from any path; a tall, spreading 'tree', I placed the bowl on top of a tall stool to have the bowl and water just underneath some of the blooms.

This essence is like a fountain of joy in the heart, immediately uplifting and cheerful. Amongst many uses, this would be a wonderful essence to offer at weddings and other family parties. But it is also good to take when you simply wish to bring a bit of extra joy into your day!

So far these are the only two of the rhododendron essences we are releasing, but we shall see comes. Both the gardens and the island offer so many enticing blooms, doubtless there will be further 'explorings'...!

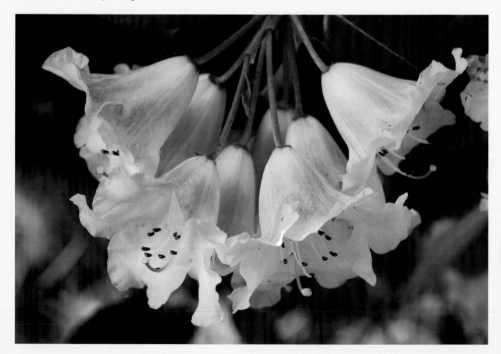

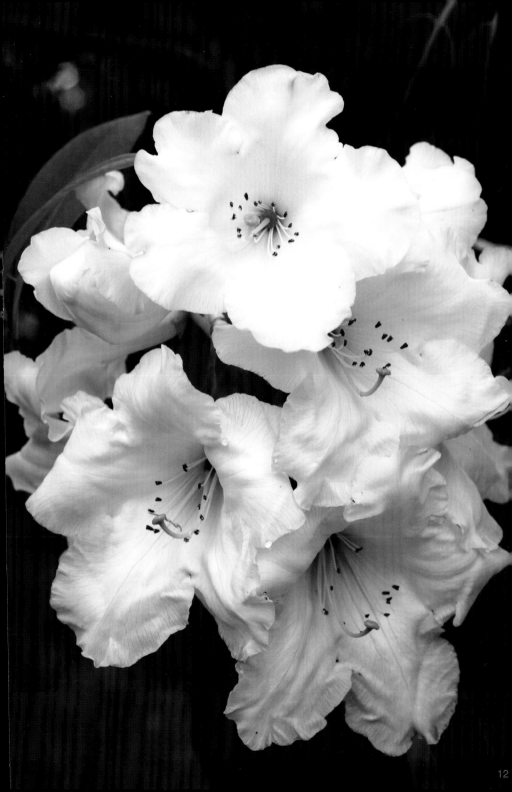

Achamore Gardens

is one of the principal destinations for visitors to Gigha, and it isn't hard to see why, especially if you visit in the peak of the blooming season in April, May or June. After the rhododendrons, azaleas and the camellias are largely past, the gardens still offer a wide variety of blooms to enjoy. The two-acre Walled Garden becomes a focus

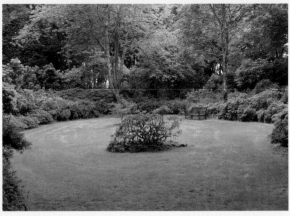

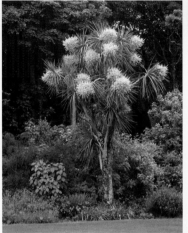

from June onwards, and even in August I counted well over a hundred different types of plants in flower across the gardens without even making a concerted effort.

The gardens are owned and maintained by the Isle of Gigha Heritage Trust, the association which was formed by the islanders for the purposes of the historic community buyout of Gigha in March 2002. They employ two full-time gardeners to look after the 52 acres, along with some part-time and occasional volunteers. These are stunning gardens, and well worth traveling to see.

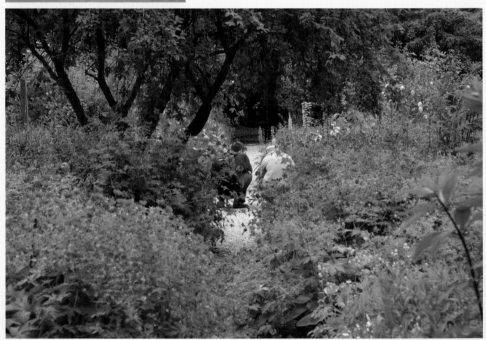

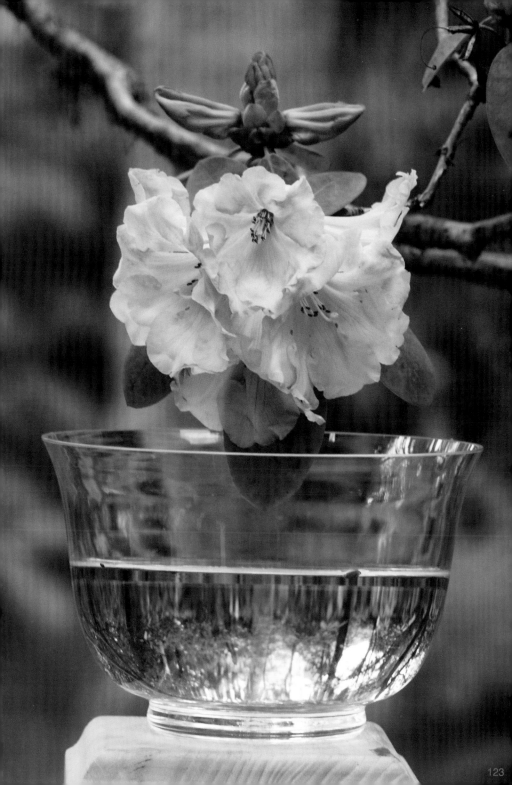

Useful Contacts and Overseas Distributors

In the UK the LTOE are available from several good outlets, including:

Ainsworths Homeopathic Pharmacy at 36 New Cavendish Street, London W1G 8UF

Helios Homeopathy Ltd. in Tunbridge Wells, Kent   www.helios.co.uk

The Psychic Piglet at 8 High Street, Glastonbury

Revital Health Food Stores in England   www.revital.co.uk

From IFER direct, either by phone or our website: **www.HealingOrchids.com**

Overseas we have a number of good distributors (and a few outlets I wish to mention):

United States:
Southern Herb Co.   www.southernherb.com   tel. 800-795-1354   (our Distributor)

Aura Visions (a shop) 20929 Ventura Blvd. #37, Woodland Hills, CA 91364

Canada:
Alypsis Inc. / Andrew Christopher   www.alypsis.ca

Japan:
Healing Essence / Junko Terayama   www.healingessence.jp

Australia & New Zealand:
Healing Orchids Australia / Jane Lindsay   www.healingorchids.com.au

Hong Kong:
The New Age Shop 7 Old Bailey Street, Soho

Austria:
SpiritLife / Brigitte Reinberger   www.SpiritLife.at

Belgium: (a shop and a website, run by Alain Wauters)
Harmonies   22 Avenue Adolphe Demeur   Bruxelles   http://users.skynet.be/fa526031

Czech Republic:
Esence pro Vas zivot, s.r.o. / Tatana Kaiserova   www.e-esence.cz

France: (where Eve Apprill has both a shop and website)
Art'Stella 66 ave. de Saint Mandé, Paris 75012   www.artstella.com

Germany:
FlowerEnergies.com / Helmut Maier who is our Distributor for Germany.

Lebensfreudeprodukte Gabriele Scheidel in Abenberg D-91183 is a licensed pharmacy which stocks the LTOE. Adalbert Scheidel knows the essences well, as does Helmut above.

Holland:
Flower Energy / Dirk Albrodt   www.flowerenergy.nl

Italy:
Spiritual Remedies   www.spiritualremedies.it

Norway:
Den Lille Arkana Youngstorget 6, Oslo 0028   www.denlillearkana.com

Spain:
La Rueda / Carmen Yates & Andrea Ramírez   www.larueda.es

Technical / Production Notes

This book is to my mind a good example of some of the beneficial ways in which technology has developed in the past couple of decades. Throughout our company's 14 years we have used Apple's computers. I will always be grateful to Steve Jobs and the people at Apple for designing and building reliable, powerful yet easy-to-use equipment. I have to admit I am looking forward to viewing this book on their iPad almost as much as I look forward to seeing the printed edition.

The book has been written using the same software I have used for page layout: Quark Xpress. I avoided Microsoft Word, as there is something about that program which to my mind is simply not conducive to creative writing. The photos have all been edited in Photohop (a program I love & would find difficult to live without), and the photo montages were created in Photoshop as well. The drawing at the bottom of this page was created using SketchUp.

The photos have all been taken with Nikon cameras over the past 11 years. I went digital when the D1X was brought out in the summer of 2001. Back then 5.4 million pixel images seemed pretty good, certainly enough to draw me away from the inconveniences presented by film. Something subtle is lost in that transition, but the ease of shooting digital more than makes up for it in my view. Many of the photos I have taken in the past 5 years were shot with the D2X, and I now use a D3X. The black background in most of the photos was achieved using a good black cloth draped behind the orchid, with the resulting black then tweaked in Photoshop.

Nearly all of the photos in the book are ones I have taken. There are eight exceptions: page 14 (aerial); page 16's photo of Tanmaya, Arthur & Christine was taken by Kathrin Bateman of Fox Mountain; page 21 (Peter, Heather); page 23 (Dominic); page 19's photo was taken by a very cold Emma Dennis; page 94's photo of me and Günther Ludwig was taken by Inge Ludwig; and the photo of me on the drums on page 95 was taken by my late schoolteacher Mr. Winton.

The Orchid Sanctuary

Our present greenhouse has suited our essence-making needs well, but it is a bit cramped if I wish to bring visitors inside to meet the orchids. So I have drawn up plans for a greenhouse next to our existing one, which would be substantially larger, to create one of the finest publicly-viewable orchid collections in Scotland. The aim is to help educate people about the tremendous diversity of orchids in general, and about orchid conservation issues. For those wishing to learn about their energetic qualities, this will also be available of course. But most people only know of orchids by what they see in the supermarkets, and I would like to help change that. I hope to build the new greenhouse in 2011, providing we can get the funding in place. Should anyone wish to learn more, please feel free to contact me by phone or email; or you could just knock on the door if you happen to be passing by...

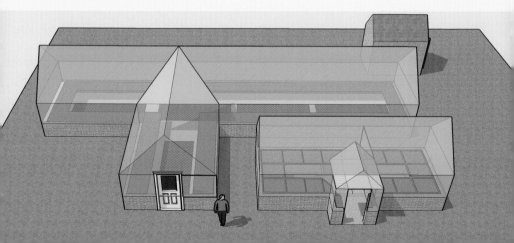

Acknowledgements

A project like the creation of the Living Tree Orchid Essences has involved many people over the years, and I wish to take the opportunity to express my appreciation to some of them.

As I have said earlier, the LTOE would not have come into being were it not for Heather DeCam participating in the making of the essences with me not long after I had started doing so. Her light, warmth & humour are a blessing to all who know her. Heather's husband Pierre-Loup helped us to understand important aspects of chemistry in relation to the essences, and also helped me with his eye for design when we decided to produce photographic labels for each of the essences. Pierre-Loup also never grumbled when his wife had to spend evenings away at the Living Tree helping to make a new orchid essence. To both of them, I send my deepest thanks.

Shabd-sangeet Khalsa has had more impact on current developments in flower essence making than most people will know about. Co-founding the Alaskan Flower Essence Project and nursing it through the first 8 years of its activity was no mean feat; she then created her own line of the Dancing Light Orchid Essences, and demonstrated unequivocally the value of making essences with orchids raised within a greenhouse environment. And through her passion for the plants themselves, she inspired my interest in orchids. I owe her a great debt of gratitude.

The dialogues with Peter Tadd about the qualities of the orchid essences were deeply enriching, and thought-provoking, and enabled me to consider the orchids with far deeper respect than would have otherwise have been the case.

The numerous friends who have been customers of IFER's over the years now are too many to list here, but I must thank Liz Kinsey for having introduced IFER to Adrian back in 1997. Like Adrian, Liz is a (very fine) homeopath who also uses essences, and has been a good friend this past decade and more. My deep gratitude of course to Dr. Adrian Brito-Babapulle, who brought whole new dimensions of understanding to working with the orchid essences, and who has become a good friend in the process.

I would also like to say my thanks to the people at Miron Glass in Switzerland for their work and research in making the finest bottles we know of for storing our mother tinctures.

View of Kintyre from the southeast shore of Gigha

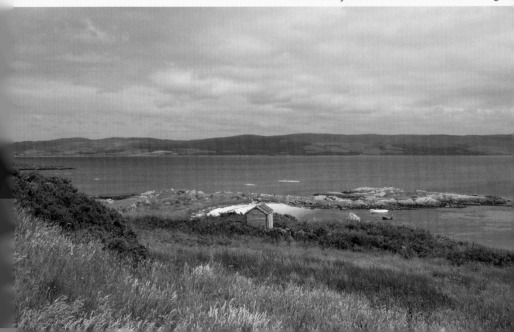

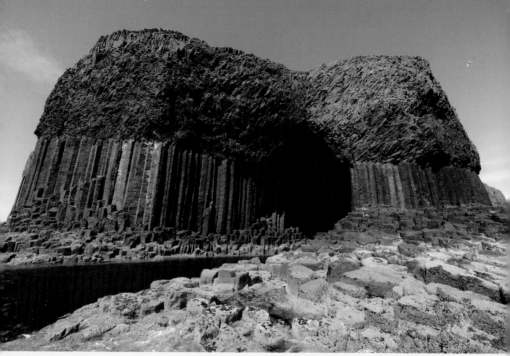

The island of Staffa with the majestic Fingal's Cave is just over 2 hours from Gigha by boat when the weather is calm. One of the geological wonders of Scotland, it inspired Felix Mendelssohn's Hebrides Overture when he visited the island in 1829. I took this photo from the shore on my second trip there, in July 2009.

IFER has always been blessed with wonderful staff, and this continues in the present. Rhona Martin brings both insight and great humour; Jennifer Brown is a terrific bookkeeper; June Watson is lovely and calm in the bottling room; while I mustn't let Rona Allan know just how valuable she is here in the office - but our customers will know in any case. Jennifer and Rona's mother Mary Allan was a great help to me in the first few years after I moved to Gigha, while Tracey McSporran helps ensure that Achamore House is a welcoming and well-run B&B.

I have the good fortune to have as my parents two of the most remarkable people I know. Both my mother and father are deeply thoughtful, conscientious, and generous. In a rare scolding when I was young, my mother chided me for not having performed a chore properly: "Any job worth doing is worth doing well!" I have approached my work with the orchid essences, and photography, and in writing this book with that thought in mind. And one day when I was nine I asked my father if the best job was the one that paid the most money. "No", he replied, "it is the one you find most meaningful, and which might also leave the world a somewhat better place than before." I believe I took this notion to heart rather more fully than he intended. But I hope they will both enjoy seeing this book, which (for me) is the result of fusing both notions in my life. My parents have shown each of their children great love; and my three children (each of whom I am immensely proud of) are very lucky to have such grandparents.

One year ago today a beautiful and very, very funny Scottish dairy farmer was mad enough to marry an odd fellow from California who makes orchid essences. I have shown the ardour of my love this winter by disappearing into my office to write this book. Emma's forbearance has been remarkable. My seminar guests have had the good fortune of meeting Emma; they know what an extraordinary woman she is, and what a lucky man I am in having married her.

- Achamore House, Isle of Gigha, March 14th 2010

Afterword

The first of the Living Tree Orchid Essences was made in September 1998, three years after our flower essence business started. The purpose of the International Flower Essence Repertoire (IFER) was the importing and distribution of the finest flower essences from around the world. We carried a few established ranges from the UK, but our focus was on helping the very best quality ranges from abroad to reach the UK market with integrity. In this capacity IFER has represented some 24 different ranges over the years since December 1995, when we were appointed as UK Distributor for the Petite Fleur Essences of Texas.

In order to help therapists and members of the public appreciate and understand how to use the various ranges we carried, IFER also began a program of weekend workshops at our premises, the Living Tree in Milland, near Liphook in Hampshire, England. These were taught by the various essence makers whose lines we represented. That we would begin producing our own line of essences was in those first few years completely unforeseen, and was indeed unexpected when it did begin to happen. But there was also a great benefit for me in hosting these numerous workshops, as the strengths (and weaknesses) of the various essence making approaches could be reflected upon; it was for me not unlike attending a post-graduate University of Flower Essences. Our essence-making process is a result of that long process and is, I believe, a good one. It has the merit of not only not harming or stressing the plants but also enables the essence to be as free as possible from the emotional and energetic 'footprint' of the essence makers. Should anyone have any questions relating to our essence making procedure, I am only too happy to share further about it - although the description provided in this book does relay all the salient details.

SSK once mentioned to me that her initial reluctance to make essences with greenhouse grown orchids disappeared when she realized that these beings - the orchids - were in our greenhouses as volunteers, that they positively *wanted* to work with us in this manner. That has been what I have found as well over the past eleven years. The greenhouse is a magical space; if you get the chance to visit Gigha, be sure to ask to experience this for yourself. I am in the greenhouse usually at least an hour a day, which is always very special. Caring for the orchids is like spending time with old friends. Stay in Achamore House for a night or two and see for yourself... I'm always happy to show our guests the very special space which is the home to our orchids.

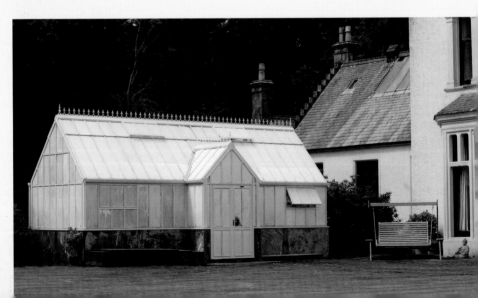